BURSTING THE BUBBLE

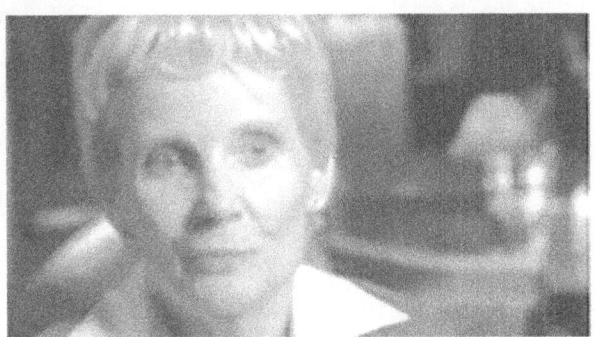

Mary Ada Murphy

Bursting the Bubble
The Tortured Life and Untimely Death of David Vetter

Mary Ada Murphy
Raymond J. Lawrence

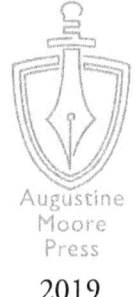

Augustine
Moore
Press

2019

© 2019 Mary Ada Murphy and Raymond J. Lawrence

All rights reserved.

Augustine Moore Press, LLC
432 West 47th Street Suite 2W
New York, NY 10036

Publisher's Cataloging-in-Publication data

Names: Lawrence, Raymond J., editor, author / Murphy, Mary Ada, author

Title: Bursting the Bubble: The Tortured Life and Untimely Death of David Vetter / Mary Ada Murphy and Raymond J. Lawrence.

Description: Includes bibliographical references and index | New York, NY: Augustine Moore Press, New York, NY

Identifiers: ISBN-13: 978-0-578-71722-7
Subjects: The case of David Phillip Vetter

Classification: Nonfiction > Biography & Autobiography > General, Nonfiction > Biography & Autobiography > Social Scientists & Psychologists

Cover by Lauren Kuo | Layout by Krista Argiropolis

Front cover, top photo: David Vetter; bottom photo: William T. Shearer, M.D, Ph.D, Mary Ada Murphy, David Vetter.

Back cover: David Vetter and Mary Ada Murphy

Inside photo of Mary Ada Murphy courtesy of American Experience/WGBH Educational Foundation.

Dedicated to DAVID PHILLIP VETTER
September 21, 1971–February 22, 1984

who was no volunteer but rather a victim
though hardly more than a child

he bore his cross with grace and wisdom

TABLE OF CONTENTS

Acronyms xi
Principals xiii
Preface xv
My Perspective on the David Vetter Case xix
1. The End—The Beginning 1
2. Age Three—The Happy Time 4
3. Age Four—David Meets Friend Number Two 16
4. How and Why 29
5. Age Four—David Gains Knowledge 34
6. The Space Suit 45
7. David Enters Grade One 63
8. The Seven-Year-Old Playwright 77
9. Looking Out from the Isolator 83
10. Seven Years in the Bubble 88
11. Age Eight—The Beginning
    of the End 95
12. The Three Alternatives 104
13. St. Jude 115
14. The Three Doctors Return 131
15. Resignation and Despair 148
16. Age Ten—David is Discharged
    from the Hospital 161
17. Eleven—The Age of Reason 175
18. A Cockroach and
    Exploding Turtles 189
19. The Transplant 203
20. The ER 220
21. Two Weeks Out of the Bubble 231

22. The Funeral 253
23. Aftermath 260
Acknowledgments 273
About the Author 275
About the Editor 276

ACRONYMS

BCM	Baylor College of Medicine
CDP	Center for Developmental Pediatrics (Meyer Center) St. Luke's Episcopal Hospital/Texas Children's Hospital
CRC	Clinical Research Center
ETO	Ethylene oxide gas
CDP	A common area in the Pediatrics Department in Texas Children's Hospital
MBIS	Mobile Biological Isolation System (space suit)
NASA	National Aeronautics and Space Administration
PVC	Polyvinylchloride (bubble-skin material)
SCID	Severe Combined Immune Deficiency
TCH	Texas Children's Hospital

PRINCIPALS

The Vetter Family

David Phillip	b. Sept. 21, 1971/ d. Feb. 22, 1984
David Joseph, Sr.	David's father
Carol Ann	David's mother
Katherine	David's sister b. April 14, 1968
David Joseph, Jr.	David's brother b. May 1970 / d. Nov. 1970

Ralph Feigin, M.D.	Chairman, Department of Pediatrics, Baylor College of Medicine; physician-in-chief, TCH
Nancy LaFevers, M.A.	Speech and language therapist,
Tom Langford	Hospital chief electrician
H. Barry Molish, Ph.D.	Associate Professor, Department of Pediatrics, BCM, and Director, Psychological Services, TCH/St. Luke's
John R. Montgomery, M.D.	Professor, Department of Pediatrics, PMC, and David's physician until March 1984
Mary Ada Murphy, Ph.D.	Child Psychologist at Baylor College of Medicine and author
Shawn Murphy	David's friend in Conroe
Buford Nichols, M.D.	Professor, Department of Pediatrics, BCM, and David's physician, March 1974 to September 1978
Elizabeth Pollard, L.V.N.	David and his brother's nurse for their entire lives
Elaine Potts, R.D.	Head Nutritionist, CRC
Arden Richardson	Conroe Independent School District
Bette Robertson, R.N.	Back up nurse, November 1979 to March 1981

Andrew Rozelle	David's friend in Houston
William T. Shearer, M.D., Ph.D.	Professor, Department of Pediatrics and Microbiology and Immunology, BCM; and Director, Center for Allergy and Immunological Disorders, TCH, from September 1978
Mary Ann South, M.D.	Professor, Department of Pediatrics, BCM, and David's physician until Summer 1983.
Susan Thurber, R.P.T.	Physical Therapist, CDP
Jackie Vogel, M.A.	Director, Child Life/Play Therapy, TCH
Raphael Wilson, Ph.D.	Professor, Department of Pediatrics, David's godfather, Gnotobiologist

PREFACE

I do not think that a baby born today with Severe Combined Immune Deficiency (SCID) would suffer the isolation that the so-called Bubble Boy, David Vetter, suffered for twelve years until his death in 1984. The reasons for this are multiple. One reason is that genetic counseling is far more sophisticated than it was in the last quarter of the 20th Century and potential parents can avoid bearing a child who could develop SCID. If a child is born with SCID and it is diagnosed within the first six months after birth, there are some powerful treatment options including bone marrow transplantation. David Vetter's sister was a donor of bone marrow for David, but it was not successful for a variety of reasons. In addition, there are now genetic therapies available that are promising. Ironically, though, in some early research trials of human subjects using genetic therapy nearly half of the research subjects developed leukemia. Luckily, the cohort was a small one of a dozen human subjects and the study was halted. SCID occurs in one out of 100,000 births, and many of those are found in populations with less than optimal medical diagnoses and care and die within a year for failure to thrive (G. Aloj, et al., 2012).

Another reason that a child probably would not live in isolation for so long is precisely the reason that Mary Murphy and Raymond Lawrence point out: the process of isolation and raising a child in isolation is an ethical quagmire. David Vetter's physicians could and did argue that what they provided was non-curative treatment that bought time to find a curative one, making the isolation hopefully unnecessary one day. The problem with this is twofold. First, when would that day come? How much of the burden of isolation was worth whatever the hoped-for benefit might have been? But the other ethical issue that was troubling is that the process of non-curative treatment morphed to become research. David Vetter was on the one hand a patient and on the other hand a research subject, and a captive one at that. I have read both the Murphy and Lawrence manuscripts, and I do not remember seeing anything about a research review board overseeing the observational research performed by the physicians and scientists involved with David Vetter. In 1974, Congress passed the National Research Act, which established the Institution Review Board (IRB), the local committee that oversees research done within an organization involving human subjects. I do not see that there was any involvement by such a board in this case. I am sure that members of an IRB would have raised significant questions about such a project. In addition, once such a project began it would have been difficult to stop it. Eventually it was stopped and David Vetter died. Was there really a fully informed consent process with David Vetter's parents? When David was older was he given the information he really deserved and, if he could not give consent legally, could he have voiced his assent or refusal? Murphy makes it clear that David did want out. Very badly he wanted out.

Perhaps I am more optimistic than I ought to be. Perhaps an IRB would not have brought the questions we might have today or that the chaplains and others had in David Vetter's day. I was in graduate school in doctoral studies from 1976 until 1981 at Princeton Theological Seminary and Princeton University. At the university I studied with Paul Ramsey, one of the pioneers of modern medical ethics. While I was vaguely aware of David Vetter in those days, and certainly aware when he died in 1984, I do not remember any real discussion about the ethical questions involved in his situation. There might have been some discussion, but if there was I was not privy to it. This is particularly striking because Ramsey first began his thinking about medical ethics on the question of children as human research subjects.

Human subject research must always be conscious of the question of the balance between the needs and protection of the patient and the needs of research. It always pits the potential of future good against the immediate good of patient care and patient protection. Making patients into research subjects can soil the sanctity of the caring relationship between patient and physician. This is not a new idea. As early as 1907, William Osler delivered a lecture, "The Evolution of the Idea of Experiment in Medicine." He made his concern and warning about human subject research by physicians very clear: "Absolute safety and full consent are conditions which make such tests allowable. We have no right to use patients entrusted to our care for the purpose of experimentation unless direct benefit of the individual is likely to follow. Risk to the individual may be taken only with his consent and full knowledge of the circumstances."

Were Osler's dictum and the principles of human research subject protections considered in the case of David Vetter? You have before you the Murphy memoir and Lawrence's critique. Let the reader be the judge.

Brian H. Childs, M.Div., Ph.D.
Professor of Bioethics and Professionalism
Mercer University School of Medicine
Columbus / Macon / Savannah, Georgia

References

Aloj, G. et al. (2012). Severe Combined Immunodeficiencies: New and Old Scenarios. *International Review of Immunology.* 31:1.

Osler, W. (1907). The Evolution of the Idea of Experiment in Medicine. *Transactions of the Congress of American Physicians and Surgeons*, v. 7, 1-8.

MY PERSPECTIVE ON THE DAVID VETTER CASE

by Raymond J. Lawrence

Mary Ada Murphy was the principal caretaker of David Vetter, the Bubble Boy of Houston, who died in 1984 at age twelve and a half. The story of his experience of living perpetually in a sterile chamber has not up to this point been told. His experience was unique in human history. We can hope such an experiment will never be repeated. From the very beginning until now the public has been fed the propaganda of a happy Bubble Boy, but Mary Murphy tells us otherwise. At this late date it will be difficult—though perhaps not impossible—either to corroborate or to refute Mary's account. Many of the key witnesses are dead, and many of the actors prefer that the actual story of David's experience be left in his grave, assigned to oblivion.

II

The great twentieth century German theologian, Paul Tillich, said in the 1930s, in a discussion with Christian authorities of the rise of Adolf Hitler as a political leader, that Hitler did not qualify as an antichrist figure in Christian tradition because he lacked one essential element: the appearance of goodness. To qualify as quintessential evil one must have the appearance of goodness. The infamous Bubble Boy Case was an evil medical project, and the fact that it was presented to the world as a humanitarian rescue with all the aura of goodness made it trenchantly evil. The Bubble Boy project explicitly denigrated the importance of a full social existence, including human physical contact, and by extension it denigrated the place of sexuality in the human experience. Remarkably, or perhaps not so remarkably, this denigration seems to have functioned mostly at an unconscious level.

In the Bubble Boy case medicine was said to have saved from certain death a child suffering from Severe Combined Immune Deficiency (SCID) by placing him in a sterile chamber where he would be protected from all the many microorganisms that threatened to kill him. Once safely ensconced in the plastic bubble (polyvinylchloride or PVC, essentially a large balloon), a search was begun to find closely matched bone marrow that could be transplanted in the patient. The bone marrow transplant would theoretically jump-start the patient's own immune system and allow the patient safely to exit the bubble and live a normal social life with other beings. As it turned out, however, no compatible bone marrow was ever found. But even worse, no viable exit strategy was projected for the patient. Even more foreboding, the medical team was satisfied that permanent life in the sterile chamber was little more than an inconvenience.

In the beginning of this project there was said to be every hope of finding the appropriate bone marrow match that would reconstruct the patient's immune system, allowing him to exit the sterile chamber and survive in the outside world with its plethora of lethal bacteria and viruses. The search may well have been diligent. But from the medical team's perspective, the search was not a matter of utmost urgency. The medical team's fallback position was that the child, if necessary, could live his entire life in the bubble. As the medical team said, he was otherwise healthy and had "a good mind," and they viewed such confinement as comparable to being dependent on an iron lung, a facile comparison. It was said by the medical team leader that the patient could live a productive life in the sterile chamber "for eighty years" if necessary. But the bubble was not comparable to an iron lung. The bubble prohibited absolutely any tactile human contact or even any contact with unfiltered air. This restriction prohibited the patient from anything resembling a social existence as one human being among others. As the patient matured he came to be aware of his strange, unique and isolated existence. He complained that he was brought into the world and treated as if he were "a wild animal in a cage." Data suggest that as the years passed he was slowly growing mad.

It appeared very early on that the patient might be trapped for life in the sterile chamber. But worse, the scientists and physicians who put him there were content—even blasé—about that possibility. For the decision-makers, there was no rush. I contend that they—consciously or unconsciously— harbored a hidden agenda. They were intent on nurturing a human being untouched by sin, and specifically the sin of sex, and that this covert vision explains their cavalier attitude toward the question of whether the patient would ever be able to leave the sterile chamber.

No one in the medical community has yet come clean to confess that this project was demonic at its core, should never have been carried out in the first place, and must never be repeated. Subsequent to the death of the patient in 1984, all we have heard in the public discourse from the physicians and scientists responsible is that there is no longer a need to do what was done in this case because we now have found a way to treat and cure the SCID syndrome. While true, that is not enough. It must be said openly that medicine must never again subject a human being involuntarily and permanently to such deprivation.

A failure of self-reflection on the part of virtually the entire medical community has resulted in tacit retrospective approval of the actions of the medical team in placing this newborn infant in the sterile chamber for life. The medical community at large originally neglected to consider the consequences of the possible failure to find a cure for the missing immune system. This posture permitted the medical team to take a peculiarly glib and nonchalant attitude toward the implications of life in permanent isolation, and even to tolerate an announcement by the team that they would do it again if the same circumstances arose. Such was their hubris. All the while, the entire medical community looked the other way. There was in the medical team a gross failure to consider the implications of total and permanent deprivation of physical human contact for a lifetime.

The medical team at the onset of this case consisted of two physicians, John R. Montgomery and Mary Ann South, and a Ph.D. gnotobiologist and immunologist, Raphael Wilson. (Gnotobiology comprises the study of living beings raised in germ-free environments.) Wilson was the putative team leader and the most enthusiastic of the three. As Mary Ann South said, "He just swept us along with his enthusiasm… [saying] 'We can do it. We can do it.'" There was even an innuendo of glee about this scientific project that was chilling. Gossip in the hospital reported that subsequent to David's safe delivery Wilson was excitedly telling his friends in the hospital, "I got my baby!" Wilson was a monk in the Order of the Holy Cross. His cavalier claim that the patient, with a good mind and body, could if required do well permanently in the sterile chamber, suggests that Wilson saw the sterile chamber, not as a grim and tragic form of permanent imprisonment, but as some kind of nouveau monk's cell where the patient could find sexual purity and religious salvation.

For more than twelve years the patient, or should we say this object of scientific experiment, endured his absolute isolation, increasingly aware that he was imprisoned for life. As the credulous public was fed a sanguine tale about this boy who had been saved by modern medicine, the patient himself gradually became more and more despairing. When the patient was about eight years old the medical experts did finally confirm privately that the likely choices for him were indeed life permanently trapped in the bubble or death outside, and that they had nothing else to offer him. By then the original medical team had departed Houston and a new team was in place.

The root of the medical community's dysfunction in the Bubble Boy case was professional loyalty. Physicians and scientists are reluctant to challenge one another privately or publicly. Once the original medical team had departed, when David was about five years old, the succeeding medical teams were reluctant to criticize the decisions of the original team. This professional loyalty stymied both clear thinking and decisive action. In addition to professional loyalty, the growing person of David Vetter himself was an increasing concern. He was after all a human being, even if he felt like he was a rat in a cage. A further inhibition of any candid discussion of David's plight was the inchoate dread of legal action by the family. Each of these issues hobbled the medical treatment of David from the very beginning.

This story is unique in human history. It is haunting. It should be told. I contend that it was a scientific experiment covertly driven by a religious ideology valuing sexual purity. It should never have been undertaken. It should never be repeated.

Remarkably, a medical conference was held in Houston in 1977 bearing the theme, "Research in Children." Eleven of the featured speakers were medical experts residing in Houston. The Chicago ethicist Kenneth Vaux, who was also quite familiar with the Bubble Boy case, was in attendance. No mention was made in the conference of the then six-year-old David Vetter, even though the conference was hardly more than a bicycle ride away from David's sterile prison. Another case of the emperor's new clothes.

III

The Bubble Boy was David Vetter, the third child of a twenty-something Catholic couple from Conroe, Texas, forty miles north of Houston. David had a sister, older by three years. He had a brother, also named David, who himself had died of SCID at seven months of age. Ten months after the death of the first David the mother gave birth to the second David whose life was lived in the bubble.

The first David was brought to Texas Children's Hospital (TCH) in grave condition and died there around Thanksgiving, 1970. Coincidentally, a gnotobiological and immunological medical team was already in place at TCH, led by Raphael Wilson, Ph.D. The team was seeking potential patients. They approached the Vetter family immediately after the death of their first son and informed them of the resources they had to offer. Were the grieving parents to give birth to another boy with the SCID syndrome, the hospital had in place the means to keep him alive while waiting for a cure. (Genetically, the SCID syndrome affects only males, of which fifty percent are symptomatic.) The bubble was conceived before David himself was. Barely one month after burying her first son, Carol Ann Vetter was pregnant with her third child. Amniocentesis later determined that the fetus was male. Whether he was carrying the SCID syndrome could not be determined in the womb. Thus the sterile chamber was constructed and prepared for the possibility of the infant carrying the syndrome. This practicing Catholic couple never considered abortion, and the motivation of the quick pregnancy was the prospect of treatment if the infant was a carrier of SCID. The infant was delivered by Caesarian section in order to thwart exposure of organisms in the birth canal. The obstetric team stood still for fifteen minutes prior to delivery in order to let any dust settle. They did not speak, but communicated only with hand signals. The infant was in a matter of seconds placed directly into the bubble without any evidence of contamination. Some days later he was found to be without a thymus gland, and therefore was determined in fact to be a carrier of the SCID syndrome. The medical team then instituted a search to find an appropriate donor match that might offer the option of a bone marrow transplant. No appropriate match was found in the twelve-year search.

IV

Serendipitously, I came to know about and finally to know personally David Vetter. David was born September 21, 1971, and died February 22, 1984. Many of the key actors are already deceased. Like much in life, both my knowing David and knowing about him his entire life was the result of a number of odd convergences. I simply happened to be in the right—or wrong—place at the right time. Ultimately, I came to know the larger story of this case probably as well as anyone still living.

It all started for me in the early 1970s. I was on the chaplaincy staff for Texas Children's/St Luke's Episcopal Hospital in Houston. In 1973 I was appointed interim department head, and in that capacity I eventually visited David for the first time. An entire nurses' station was given over to David. He and the bubble itself were very high maintenance, requiring constant surveillance. Any small penetration of the sterile chamber or failure of the blowers was a potential threat to David's life. The blowers provided positive air pressure so that small breaks would force air out until repairs could be made. A failure of the blowers in creating positive pressure, keeping the bubble inflated, would be a threat to David's life. While I visited him in my capacity as Director of Pastoral Care, I was not in any real sense his chaplain. It was made clear to me that Raphael Wilson, gnotobiologist and medical team leader, functioned also as his religious advisor and chaplain. Both David's family and Wilson were Roman Catholics. Wilson was a monk, and the family bonded strongly with him. He had baptized David with sterilized holy water immediately at his birth. By the time I met David he was already three years old and in the process of learning the catechism. Wilson was wearing two hats, which created a genuine conflict of interest.

I was troubled by David's predicament at first sight. It was immediately clear to me that he was not going to be a boy like others. I could identity with some of the other professionals who visited him, and who reported being speechless and horrified to witness a human being trapped indefinitely in a sterile chamber. As he grew, I became more troubled. My heart went out to him. I felt that he could not tolerate such an existence for the long term. But the medical team declared themselves to be reconciled to and indeed even sanguine about the inconvenient possibility that he would have to remain indefinitely in the bubble.

In the winter of 1975, when David was three-and-a-half years old, I made a daring proposal to the medical team which was quickly and generously accepted, somewhat to my surprise. I proposed an in-house ethical case conference on the case. I approached Drs. Wilson and Montgomery personally, and they each agreed without hesitation to support it. Coincidentally, at that time the Episcopal clergyman and world-renown ethicist, Dr. Joseph Fletcher, was temporarily in residence for several months at the nearby Institute of Religion. I contacted Joe, whom I already knew, and he readily agreed to serve as consultant to such an ethical case review of David.

When the appointed time arrived, at noon on February 26, 1975, there were about thirty persons participating: doctors, nurses, chaplains, administrators, psychologists, and public relations personnel. It was, of course a closed meeting. Only select hospital staff was permitted to attend. The meeting opened with Raphael Wilson's very long and self-confident account of how David came to be in his sterile chamber, followed by his prognosis. It was exceedingly upbeat. The medical team hoped to find a cure and to reconstitute his immune system, but if they failed, David could live "eighty years" in the bubble if necessary. Dr. Montgomery then added his equally positive assessment. The party line was that David was doing extremely well, and there was no anxiety about how long he would have to wait for a possible cure to be found. The medical team was seeking persons with comparable or matching bone marrow, with whom they might request a transplant that would jumpstart David's non-functioning immune system. After three years they had had no success in their search for a matching donor.

Though the typed transcript of the ethical case conference does not reveal this, the almost two-hour conference deteriorated into emotional conflict when some of my fellow chaplains present and I questioned how long David could be expected to tolerate his imprisonment in the sterile chamber. The medical team became defensive. I am sure that they felt unjustly ambushed. They seemed taken aback that anyone would dare to think that continuing life in the sterile chamber was anything more than a serious inconvenience. Chaplain Robert Main, speaking for the chaplains' office as a whole, voiced the view that David would not live past puberty in the bubble, that his hormones would lead him to break out. This prognosis drew argument, defensiveness, hard feelings and even tears. The physicians responded angrily. The conference ended on a sour note. Some of the women left crying. The serious and reflective discussion that I hoped for did not materialize. Joseph Fletcher commented in a kind of benediction that the parents were wrong to bring a child to term whose prognosis for SCID was fifty-fifty. Now that David was alive the next problematic question, he added, is whether to permit David to act in such a way as to commit suicide, such as breaking out of the bubble. Fletcher indicated that his judgment was that he should have that right, although age was a constraining factor. And finally, Fletcher summed up by saying that David may very well say ultimately, "Alright, you know the flame is now no longer worth the candle." And that was in fact the conclusion that David himself seemed to come to at age nine. But Montgomery got in the last word, stating that he would willingly do this case over again with another child or with many other children.

While the case conference was far from satisfactory and resulted in unfortunate polarization, it was arguably useful in that it became in fact an accurate prognosticator of what was to come in the years ahead. As he matured, David became increasingly troubled and more difficult to control. He wanted out of his sterile prison, and at the same time he was panicked about living outside where he would be assaulted by lethal organisms. He was very intelligent. As he matured he came to know very well his likely fate: continuing life in his sterile prison or death.

As reported by Evelyn Nelson McMillan, Raphael Wilson was quoted in the popular American Medical Association journal, *Today's Health*, as urging both hospital staff and the Vetter family never to talk to David in terms of "when you get out." This is further evidence of Wilson's propensity to see the sterile chamber as a potentially permanent dwelling.

The ethical case conference did not help my standing in the hospital. I was terminated abruptly several months later, in July, allegedly for publishing an academic paper (on another subject!) without hospital permission. I never saw David again.

A most unlikely turn of events, however, put me back in contact with David, though indirectly. The hospital electrician, Tom Langford, and I had bought a small apartment complex years earlier, and Tom was wanting to sell his share of the partnership. He interested a fellow hospital employee, Mary Ada Murphy, to buy his interest in the building. Mary was a psychologist in the process of completing her Ph.D., focusing on childhood development. Mary had likely become friendly with Langford from his frequent visits with David. He would typically bring his bag lunch up to David's bubble and spend time with him. Langford was frequently called upon to do maintenance on the sterile chamber, which was a Rube Goldberg contraption. He and David eventually became very close.

Mary's hospital office, where she gave psychological tests to children, was very close to David and his bubble. But she had not met him until he was three years old and, in fact, was negatively disposed in general to the Bubble Boy project. However, the Director for Psychological service, Dr. Barry Molish, assigned her the task of testing David psychologically at age three. Eventually—and unofficially—she effectively became David's "hospital mother." She was actually present at the infamous Ethical Case Conference that I convened, but at the time I did not know her, never having met her personally. So Mary bought Langford's share of the apartment project and joined this small business venture with me. Subsequently, we became close friends and remained so for more than three decades, for the rest of Mary's life. Sometime about 2010 she developed Alzheimer's and moved to the Philippines to be cared for by her widowed daughter-in-law. All my subsequent attempts to locate her in the Philippines were for naught. Notice of her death came to me from a third party without specifics regarding cause, date, or place of her death. Data posted on the Internet indicated that she died in August, 2013.

What I learned about David subsequent to July 1975, I learned directly from Mary Murphy or from the typescripts she wrote in the years following David's death.

V

As Mary tells it, she first met David September 25, 1974, at his family home. He was three. She was sent to give him a psychological test, accompanied by the director of her department, Barry Molish, Ph.D. A duplicate sterile chamber had just been constructed at the family home, and he was beginning a regimen of spending about half his time at home. Mary bonded with David very quickly. She was that kind of person. She talked straight, exuded warmth, and was quietly self-confident. David expressed curiosity to her about the leaves on a tree he observed out his window. His sister had tried to pick one, but could not reach it. So Mary went out in the rain, with an umbrella that the wind upended, and a bit drenched, brought in a small branch with leaves for David to see up close. Mary became "the lady who brought me the leaf." On their next encounter, at the hospital, David said, "Lady, you brought me the leaf. Now bring me little cars," specifying that their doors had to open, including "the front door," as he called the hood.

Later, during a period when David was resident in the hospital, he was refusing to cooperate with the medical staff—as was often the case—who were trying to entice him to enter his larger newly added playroom. He preferred to remain in his old sleeping quarters. It seems he had bumped his head in attempting to climb down out of the smaller sleeping chamber and refused to try again. Reporters and photographers had arrived to write the story of the Bubble Boy entering his new expanded living quarters. But they left empty handed. Days later, Mary was informed of David's recalcitrance, and she tricked him by bringing in a bowl of goldfish for him to see. She cleverly positioned herself at the far end of the new playroom. David had never seen such a thing as live fish before, and he came out of his sleeping quarters and into the far end of the playroom in a flash. His interest in goldfish, tropical fish, and live shrimp continued all his life, and later he was even able to care for them, or rather to direct their care, from inside his bubble. More importantly, David gradually bonded with Mary, and profoundly so. She saw him almost every day that he was in the hospital, often remaining with him until 1:00 a.m., when he typically fell asleep. She visited him often at his home when he was ensconced there, usually on weekends and usually sleeping over. She babysat him at times in the family home so that his parents could have time off from their round-the-clock burden of maintaining him. She was with him when he died a decade later. Mary became David's principal, but unofficial medical caretaker. And she was functionally his hospital mother.

VI

By the time David was five, each of the three members of David's medical team had left or were leaving Houston for other jobs. Raphael Wilson was the last to leave. However, each of the three continued to have close contact with the family, and made occasional visits to the Vetter home to see David himself. This became a matter of serious concern for the succeeding medical teams.

Before Wilson departed Houston he approached NASA and encouraged a team of technicians there to create a space suit for David so that he could take "space walks" and see more of the world. At first glance it seemed a brilliant idea. Several engineers at NASA, specifically Bill Carmean, Paul Ferguson, and Dick Graves, generously gave considerable time and money of their own to create such a suit for David. He actually took six "space suit walks," the first when he was six years old. They were touted in the popular press, with photos, as a wonderful contribution to David's life. But, in fact, the generosity of the NASA engineers ended on something of a sour note. In spite of much time and money—and noble intentions—the space walks were more trouble than they were worth, and the physicians halted them after six walks. A major problem was that David was frightened of them. Trained all his life to be careful of germs entering his chamber, and always watching for holes or tears in the plastic, the process of entering the space suit terrified him. It took some time to entice him to get into it. Fifty minutes was the speediest entry process of the six spacesuit walks. Once in the space suit he was still quite limited. Many precautions needed to be taken. He had to be accompanied by a number of technicians and other staff. He could not be close to any sharp object. He had to be kept away from crowds, where people would stare at him as a freak, or try to touch him. The walks were monumentally difficult and labor intensive, with meager benefits. Clearly, David did enjoy certain aspects of the walks as when at home he got a chance to spray his sister, spontaneously, with a garden hose. But on balance David did not like the space walks. The public, of course, read the glowing reports about them, believing that they normalized David's life. It was quite the contrary.

David's diet for his entire life consisted mainly of baby food. He could not eat anything that was not completely sterile. This, of course, eliminated any fresh vegetable or fruit—and most of the food we normally eat. Life in the sterile chamber also prevented David from having things that most of us take for granted. It was late in his life before NASA was able to contrive a pencil that could be sterilized, and later, even an eraser. David's annual birthday parties were haunting to contemplate. While family and friends enjoyed birthday cake, ice cream, and socializing, David could only observe from inside the sterile chamber. To eat, or even to touch ice cream or cake would likely have been fatal to him.

By Mary's account David had a vivid imagination and sometimes a poetic way with words. To the woman physician whom he did not like he assigned the epithet "she," a powerful way of depersonalizing her. He assigned persons quite inventive monikers in the manner of an adult. His own mother he nicknamed "Miss Late Bird," focusing on a behavior pattern of hers. It is doubtful she ever heard him say such a thing. She would not likely have tolerated such caricatures of anyone.

As David grew older he was eventually able to use the telephone by way of the rubber gloves built into the sterile chamber's wall, and he could actually dial numbers. In addition to television, the phone became his major connection to the world outside. And unlike television, the phone offered two-way communication. He called his family and Mary at will, and often. Mary eventually assigned him the job of managing her son's small apartment building in Montrose, the artistic and countercultural section of Houston. This was educational for David, who was exposed to many actual problems of living outside the bubble. David would answer tenant complaints, call a plumber, remind tenants that they were late on their rent, and such things as that. It was also reported to hospital Administration that David was making random calls at night to Houston residents informing them that he was the famous Bubble Boy, calls that sometimes resulted in long conversations. Occasionally, a Houston resident would contact hospital administration to inquire whether the caller had actually been the Bubble Boy, or a prankster. The staff believed that it was likely David. He certainly had that kind of imagination and audacity. He was also quite self-aware, and an inveterate prankster. Hospital administration did not pursue this, blessedly allowing David a certain limited private life.

But David's life was not by any means a life of fun and pranks. He was increasingly troubled as he matured. He exhibited symptoms of deep disturbance. Staff would often find him sucking his thumb and rocking, staring into the distance even as he grew older. Staff would hear him repeating the refrain over and over, "One, two, three, four, I can't take this anymore." Nurse Dorothy Johnson said, "I would go in his room. He'd just be sitting there, staring into space. I would speak. He would reply: 'I don't want to talk. You know. Leave. Get out.' " Mary relates that David reported dreams about the King of Germs capturing him. Her rejoinder was to help him rewrite the dream's ending, in which he was the winner. David expressed the view that he should have been allowed to die at age three when he would not have known about death or what was killing him. Now, later in life, he would have to make the choice himself to remain in the bubble or leave and face death by his own choice.

All of David's sex education came either from television or adult staff persons. He had virtually no private contact with peers. And when he did, he was hardly a peer. Mary was of course, given her close relationship with David, his main sex educator. One of the first things Mary taught David was not to self-stimulate sexually or masturbate in the open, nor to perform his toileting in public, which he was still doing at the age of three. Of course David's entire existence was quite public, and establishing a measure of real privacy was near to impossible. At the most he could position himself behind draped sheets.

VII

Some curious developments about David's perceptions emerged, and have been described in published psychological literature written by Murphy herself and her colleagues. One related to David's concept of what he saw outside his hospital window. He could not be persuaded that the buildings he viewed from his windows were three-dimensional. Attempts to clarify his distortion, using play blocks and other devices, failed to persuade him otherwise. Another oddity in David's perception was that he could not be persuaded that anything existed under the surface of the earth visible to him from his window. Jackie Vogel, Director of Child Life/Play Therapy, went to great lengths to show him actual potted plants, pulling them up by their roots to demonstrate what the ground on the outside was like. But David would have none of it. Nor could David grasp what a large body of water was. It baffled him. No explanation would suffice to persuade him that there was something under the surface of a body of water. When Mary planned a trip to Singapore to see her son, David could not fathom why she was unable to avoid uncomfortable air travel and to drive the entire way over land and sea. He was adamant that the surface of the sea was as firm as the surface of the earth. In a related vein, David also became disoriented on one of the "space suit walks" that he made at his family's home. Mary noted that he could not be persuaded that his own backyard was in the back of his house. He insisted that it was across the street. What psychologists have done with these perceptual quirks, and what significance they may have, I do not know. At very least they would seem to signal that his perceptual experience, as a result of confinement to the sterile chamber, was quite singular. (See "Looking Out from the Isolator: David's Perception of the World," Mary A. Murphy and Jacqueline B. Vogel, *Journal of Developmental and Behavioral Pediatrics*, Vol. 6, No. 3, June 1985.)

VIII

Prior to the departure of Raphael Wilson in 1976, Russell J. Blattner, M.D., the physician-in-chief of TCH, demanded that Wilson dismantle the Bubble Boy project. Wilson defiantly refused. "Stop it yourself if you want," he replied. Blattner took no further action. It was one thing to put David in the sterile chamber; it was quite something else to take him out. No one was going to be put in the position of killing David. Wilson certainly knew that.

The departure of the original three members of David's medical team coincided with David's increasing awareness and intelligence. He was becoming more acutely aware of his difference from other children, and of his isolation. And he was also becoming more acutely aware of his grim fate, that he was trapped in the sterile chamber and that leaving it meant an assault by microbes that would certainly kill him.

The departure of the original team meant that a new medical team was put in place. The late Ralph D. Feigin, M.D., was named physician-in-chief of TCH in 1977, and the late William T. Shearer, M.D., Ph.D., was named director of the TCH Center for Allergy and Immunological Disorders in 1978. Shearer became David's primary physician. Feigin and Shearer became the chief decision-makers regarding David's treatment for the rest of David's life. Neither of them was beholden to the original three medical team members. However, in the eyes of the family the original three remained the final arbiters of David's treatment course.

Feigin and Shearer had come to the conclusion that a matching bone marrow donor was not likely to be found, and that some more daring and drastic choices were going to have to be made regarding David's future. Furthermore, they were fully cognizant of David's unraveling mental status. They called for psychiatric consultation from more than one expert in the field, and the results of tests and evaluations of David were not positive. He was diagnosed as depressed and psychiatrically disturbed by more than one psychiatrist. But to be sure, David himself was generally non-cooperative with most of his psychiatric interviews.

On one occasion when David heard that another psychiatrist was coming to examine him, he posted a handwritten sign on his bubble, "Get the hell out of here." His mother forced him to take it down and apologize.

Summer 1979 was the beginning of the end from Mary's perspective, as well as the perspective of some of her colleagues. David was almost eight. By the spring of 1980, the size of the bubble had to be increased yet again because of David's growth. Increasingly, cracks were discovered in the plastic sheeting. More and more complaints were registered about David's behavior. The family seemed increasingly passive and immobilized. The last of the original supporting auxiliary staff persons departed, the very sympathetic Head Nutritionist, Elaine Potts. In the summer of 1980 Feigin and Shearer concluded that David's situation was intolerable.

Shearer made an appointment with the Vetters and informed them that it was time for some risky and long shot attempts to address David's lack of immunity, such as a transplant from David's sister. The Vetters took exception to this. Supported by the original medical team, they stood firm in their resolve to wait for a cure. They elected not to risk David's life for a long shot cure. In response to this discouraging prognosis from Shearer, they made immediate contact with the three original members of the medical team.

The three came to Houston uninvited and gave Shearer and Feigin their unsought consultation. The three took the position that David should remain in the bubble until a cure was found. Montgomery offered to serve as an ongoing consultant provided he was paid a fee and travel expenses, and given six weeks notice of meetings. The meeting between the original medical team and the current medical team was tense and marked by tightly controlled hostility. The result was a standoff. Shearer was more than gracious outwardly, but he did not seek or accept further counsel from the original three. He could easily and justifiably have escorted them off the hospital property for subverting his relationship with the Vetter family. Undoubtedly, that is what he wished he could have done. The Vetters remained bonded with the original three doctors. But Shearer did not react, a tribute to his coolness under fire.

Amidst this crisis, the Vetters brought a St. Jude's medal to David and asked him to wear it, after sterilization, and to pose for a photograph. David refused. Mary and some of her colleagues were angry about this, concerned about the public innuendo of David's hopeless plight. (St. Jude is the patron saint of Lost Causes, and David was no naïf.) Inside the bubble it was relatively easy for David to refuse to cooperate. No one could lay hands on him there. His mother was about the only one who could threaten him, and she did just that. He did finally put the medal around his neck and posed for the camera as instructed. But he foiled the project with Mary's subversive guidance, slipping the medal itself inside his shirt, thwarting the entire exercise. Some years after David's death the medal was found secreted in the hem of one of the bubble's curtains.

The Vetters concurred with the original medical team and refused to agree to any experimental treatment. Shearer later countered by decreeing, appropriately, that David would no longer qualify as an inpatient of the hospital. He would be permitted two weeks residence a year for checkups, one week in the winter and one in the summer. Otherwise, David would have to be housed elsewhere, presumably at home. Thus on July 31, 1981, David, by now almost ten years old, was sent home for good. The hospital was no longer his home. But, as it turned out, neither was his family home a real home for him.

IX

In the spring of 1981, David discussed with Mary at length, and on his own initiative, the option of leaving the sterile chamber and taking his chances on a truncated life in the outside world. He knew, of course, and Mary confirmed this to him, that his prognosis would be a maximum of six months of life before some microorganism would kill him. He was anxious about dying, but he was also anxious about whether he could adjust to the different world outside. Nevertheless, he decided that he wanted to take his chances. Continuing life in the sterile chamber was intolerable. With the assistance of Mary, David began rehearsing a prepared speech that he would present to Shearer, in which he would claim the right to leave the bubble on his own initiative.

David prepared and rehearsed his speech: "Dr. Shearer, I want to discuss a serious matter. I would like some medical information about my case. I know you can't give me exact answers, but what could I expect if I came out?"

David rehearsed this speech over a couple of days in the presence of Mary. He was clearly nervous about his proposal, and about his physician's response. He then asked Mary to request an appointment with Shearer. When Shearer arrived at the appointed time, David invited him to sit on the stool typically used by visitors, as Mary stood stage right, so to speak. When Shearer demurred, David instructed him with forced bravado to "sit down." Seemingly incensed by such a peremptory command from a child patient, Shearer responded, "Children do not speak to adults that way." He remained standing. From that point all was lost. David lost his nerve. He brought up some inconsequential matters, and that was that. After Shearer left David broke down sobbing and did not recover his spirits for the rest of the day. Shortly thereafter David began his new regimen of permanent residence at his family home, with a semi-annual weeklong visit to the hospital.

In Shearer's defense, he was, according to Mary, determined to maintain a certain professional distance from David, which was arguably the physician's proper role. He was making hard decisions about David's life that he felt should not be determined by his personal feelings. As far as Mary knew, Shearer never became aware of David's aborted plan to leave the bubble and live out the brief rest of his life.

Two years later, as David was dying, Shearer then relaxed his professional role as a physician in very poignant episodes that Mary vividly recounts. He even went so far as to assist David with his toileting, a task hardly congruent with distance, or with the physician's role. Clearly Shearer loved David personally but must have felt, earlier, that he could not afford to relate to David on an informal basis.

X

In the subsequent two years Mary saw less of David. The consequences for David's being permanently at home were not positive. He had possessed a wide network of hospital employee friends. The hospital was his community. He was on the listening end to all hospital gossip. He knew patients and their prognoses. Mary was often astonished that David sometimes knew more than she did about goings-on at the hospital. At one point, when another SCID patient was admitted, the medical staff decided that it was best that David not be told of an admission of a patient with a similar diagnosis as his own, and the word was passed around to keep the information from David. But in no time at all he knew, and inquired of Mary how the patient was doing. At home David had his family and visitors, but nothing like the dynamism and variety of relationships that he had in a major medical center where he was a star patient. Furthermore, he was separated for the most part from Mary. She visited him at home many weekends, often sleeping over. And they talked often by phone. But it was not like having her so much of the time at his beck and call. David described his status at home as "caged in a dark and dreary home, surrounded by nothing." He obviously missed his hospital friends like Jackie, Potts, Dorothy, and especially Mary.

David's life at home, from age ten onward, was short-lived. He was an unspeakable burden to his family, requiring attentive twenty-four seven maintenance. He was not stimulated, and he was not happy. It was not long before David's parents threw in the towel. They informed Shearer that the status quo was intolerable. They defied the original medical team and informed Shearer that they would assent to whatever Shearer and his team would propose. Thus the plans for a long shot bone marrow transplant with David's sister were put in motion during the spring and summer of 1983, and the drawing of the marrow with the assistance of experts in the field took place in October, in Boston. Shearer and the Vetters, with David's sister, flew to Boston together. Shearer returned with marrow and injected it into David. The transplant was uneventful and seemingly successful. What followed was waiting, waiting to see what effect, if any, the procedure would have on David's immune system.

XI

In early December, David experienced symptoms: pains in his stomach, lethargy, and then mild fever. Shearer proposed, optimistically, that these were signs of David's immune system establishing itself. David had some good days followed by bad days throughout the month, but in early January his fever spiked and his pain rose to new levels. Shearer continued to treat the symptoms as if they were the result of David's body creating antibodies. This turned out to be wishful thinking. David's condition became increasingly dire. On February 7, Shearer decided his life was ebbing. He removed David from the sterile chamber, ending his twelve and a half years of isolation. For the first time in his life David was out in the world. He was treated with antibiotics and other medications. But nothing halted the destruction of his body. He died on February 22. The autopsy revealed that he had 150 tumors in his intestines. The transplant had not worked. The medical conclusion was that David had contracted mononucleosis from the transplant, organisms that could not be detected in the transplant material.

David died more like a mature man than a twelve-year-old boy. He said his goodbyes. He asked Mary to write his story. He asked Mary if she would be lonely without him. He thanked Dr. Shearer for what he had done for him. And his last words to Mary as she told him she had to rush off to teach a class, but would be right back, were, "Alright, Mary. Remember, I love you very much. Goodbye." When she returned he was no longer responsive. Mary later remembered that David had never previously said the word "goodbye" to her. It was always, "See ya."

Subsequent to David's death, Mary contemplated the task of writing a full record of her life with him as she had promised David. She discussed the matter with me, and undoubtedly others, and I gave her enthusiastic encouragement. I said that it would be a great loss to the world if the remarkable story of her relationship with David would be lost. So she did. And she took her time.

Dr. Feigin once referred to Mary as "an old hen with one chick." She accepted the metaphor without taking offense. Nor did Feigin likely mean to be offensive. The two had a very close and caring relationship. Feigin was essentially correct. Mary was old and protective. David was a fragile young chick. She found great meaning in caring for him. Certainly he was blessed to have her. She comforted him, protected him, and taught him about the world outside his bubble. She was his principal contact with reality, the world outside his artificial world. David was trapped in a man-made laboratory. My presumption is that she saved him from madness, or from an even more severe madness than what he experienced. The relationship between the two of them, vividly described in her typescript, between the old hen and the young chick, is both heartbreaking and inspiring. And it is quintessentially human. Her account is one of the great and most improbable love stories in human history.

Mary's typescript was rejected by many publishers. She finally found a publisher in Waco, Texas, in 1995, who agreed to publish it. As the book was being prepared, the Vetters came into possession of the draft. Their response was outrage. They composed a twenty-seven page, single-spaced letter to the publisher attacking Mary on multiple counts, charging her with a variety of crimes, false claims, and errors, and threats to sue. The publisher dropped the book.

My view of that imbroglio is that the Vetters were already committed to an idealized portrait of David, and Mary upset them in disclosing the unvarnished truth, as she saw it. It was understandable that the Vetters were reluctant to see their foibles and David's suffering on public display. At the same time, the Vetters were hardly portrayed by Mary as monsters. They were actually portrayed as sympathetic, regular and ordinary people for the most part, trying to do their best in an extraordinarily difficult situation. But it seems that the Vetters had already cast their lot with an idealized portrait of David, and that portrait was under threat of being dismantled by Mary.

XII

Subsequent to David's death there has been a paucity of serious public discussion of this phenomenal case of David Vetter. Dr. Allan J. Hamilton published a strong critique of the case in the March 26, 1984 edition of *Newsweek*. In 1985, the *Journal of the American Medical Association* (JAMA), published a strong critique written by me, entitled "David, the Bubble Boy, and the Boundaries of the Human." It got modest traction. Several newspapers, such as the *Dallas Morning News*, published my critique as well, in the form of an op-ed. Then the late Steve McVicker, a reporter for the tabloid *Houston Press*, published an in-depth, unbiased account of the case on April 10, 1997, with the headline "Bursting the Bubble". But that publication was limited to Houston. Then in 2001, Evelyn Nelson McMillan, wrote her master's thesis at Stanford University entitled A Bioethical Analysis of the Case of David, "The Boy in the Bubble." It is a very careful, judicious, and moving account of the case. But it is not as yet in circulation. McMillan describes the big picture and appropriately supplements my own recollections, McVicker's reporting, and Mary Murphy's own account of David's life and experience.

Barak Goodman and John Maggio then produced the "The Boy in the Bubble" for the television series, *American Experience* in 2006, a WGBH and Ark Media production. The ethicist James H. Jones was the voice of the moderator. It was the most serious and in-depth public critique of the case yet. There is need for a sequel. I was one of those interviewed for that program, along with medical and medical ethics personnel, family members, and Mary Murphy herself. Their advertising describes the story as "a tragic tale that pits ambitious doctors against a bewildered, frightened young couple."

As penetrating and useful as the program was, a sequel is called for. For one thing, the production did not go so far as to explore the sexual ideology that undergirded the ambition of the doctors. Nor has there been further exploration of that issue in the public media elsewhere.

Virtually all other reports in the public media make David out to be a heroic little boy who contributed much to medical science. There seems little public interest in the perverse motivation of the doctors who were oblivious to the implication of continuing life bereft of physical human contact. Quite sparse has been serious discussion of the dreadful predicament into which medical science placed the person of David Vetter. I am aware of no other reports documenting David's torment, or any challenge to the questionable decisions made by the original medical team.

XIII

The takeaway from this tragic saga is that physicians and scientists must keep an ear open to the humanities—ethics, philosophy, sociology, religion, and the arts—when venturing into strange new territory. Had the medical team been so attuned, the sterile chamber would likely have been seen as an excellent potential transition instrument, but not appropriate as a permanent dwelling. Medical science (so I have been told) has, since David, discovered that SCID usually can be cured with aggressive transplants within the first three months of life, without the necessity of closely matched tissue. They now have reported a 95% cure rate. Ironically, the assistant gnotobiologist on David's team, Patricia Bealmear, Ph.D., argued for doing just that when David was born. But she was overruled. If her opinion had been followed David would possibly be alive today, in his 40s. It seems that the team was generally too much enamored of the bubble and enamored of Wilson's vision of permanent life in the bubble. I suggest that the wish of team leader Raphael Wilson to create his little monastery was the snake in this Garden, and that it led directly to David Vetter's terrible death at the onset of puberty, just as I and the other chaplains predicted a decade earlier.

What was done to David should never have been done to anyone. And it should never again be done to another human being. As our scientific skills become even more effective we are likely to discover astonishing powers to direct and redirect human life in ways that trample on the essentials of basic humanity, such as the ability to relate to others physically as well as mentally. Scientific medicine should never again bring a child into being who must live permanently in isolation without human physical contact—and of course without the possibility of sexual relations of any sort, the arena of the principal hidden agenda in the David Vetter case.

XIV

Mary's own account is a touching document. It is an unsophisticated diary of an aging woman who gave a decade of her life to a doomed boy who was a victim of the SCID syndrome. She loved him deeply. It is hard to imagine what his life would have been like without her. He had many friends in the hospital, but none with whom he would spend so many days and nights, both in the hospital and at his home. Obviously, the typescript consists of Mary's perspective. Much of it is unverifiable. She likely has some distortions, errors, and faulty memories, as would anyone. Who can ever see and remember the whole truth about anything? But her vision of David and his case is a very credible and compassionate one, and I contend that it is very likely accurate at most every point. Having myself known Mary exceedingly well for more than a quarter century, I can vouch for her character and perceptiveness. She was a kindly and truthful woman. She did not deliberately hurt people. She did not exaggerate. She was far from driven by feelings of self-importance. She was quite wise. And she was disciplined. Some may wish to rebut or revise some elements of her account, or to add their own perspective, as well they should. But I believe in the final analysis Mary's account will be seen for what it is, as essentially true, if not absolutely true, and likely the clearest truth we will ever see in print about the life and death of David Vetter, the doomed boy who lived perhaps the strangest life in human history, until at age twelve and a half, bereft of an immune system, he was assaulted by pathogens and died.

XV

David Vetter was on a dreadful voyage not of his own choosing. He was a martyr to scientific medicine and popular Christian piety. His suffering must have been unspeakable. The very least the human community can do in his memory and honor is to reflect on his dreadful experience and see to it that similar abuse is not repeated on another human being.

On April 19, 2019, thirty-eight years after the bubble boy sterile chamber was constructed, the *New England Journal of Medicine* reported that scientists had found a cure for the Severe Combined Immune Deficiency (SCID) syndrome that afflicted David Vetter.

1.

THE END—THE BEGINNING

On a dreary, rainy, February afternoon in 1985, two women kneel at an unmarked grave in a Conroe, Texas cemetery.

"Carol Ann, it's been a year. Will our tears ever stop?"

"No, Mary. They can't. If they do, my son will be forgotten." There, on my knees, I remember the funeral procession moving slowly from the requiem mass to this gravesite. The route was lined with police and news media. Thousands of people stood along the road, on top of cars, and on buildings. So many people. I see their tears and hear their sobs.

Has a president died? No, they are mourning a boy. David. They don't even know his last name. From the beginning, the press knew his surname, but out of respect for the family's privacy, they never used it.

DAVID, THE BUBBLE BOY, DIES—the February 23, 1984, headline of newspapers all around the world—New York, London, Moscow, Singapore. The whole world grieved on that day.

David's confinement to a few square feet of germ-free space was hailed as a medical miracle and condemned as a triumph of biomedical technology over common sense. The astronomical cost of maintaining him in sterile isolation gave him the title "million-dollar boy."

At age twelve years and four-and-a-half months, 109 days after a bone marrow transplant and gravely ill, he was taken out of isolation and wheeled across the hall to a specially prepared sterile room. He lived fifteen more days. His conception, life, and death generated ethical issues, medical dilemmas, and political controversy.

David Phillip was the second son born to Carol Ann and David Joseph, Sr. of Conroe, Texas. Their first son, David Joseph, died at seven months of age, a victim of Severe Combined Immune Deficiency (SCID). He had had no immune system; any random germ in the air might have been fatal to him. On November 21, 1970, a week after receiving a bone marrow transplant from his two-year-old sister, Katherine, he died of pneumonia. The autopsy findings were consistent with an X-linked recessive combined immune deficiency.

After the infant's death, the two physicians who had cared for him, Drs. Mary Ann South and John Montgomery, provided the parents with genetic counseling. But no test could determine if a woman or a fetus carried the defective gene.

Doctors told Carol Ann that if the cause had been a random, sporadic mutation, there was only a one-in-ten-thousand chance of such a tragedy happening again. But if the cause were a defective X chromosome, then there was a fifty-fifty chance that any son born to her would inherit the same potentially lethal gene.

A look at family backgrounds uncovered no immune problems, but, unfortunately, the lack of males in Carol Ann's ancestry left the X-link question open. Carol Ann was one of four daughters, and her mother was an only child.

The treatment possibilities for a future affected son were discussed: A bone marrow transplant from the sister, the most likely donor, or a period (estimated at three months) in germ-free isolation to prevent infection might allow the immune system to mature and function effectively, or a matched marrow donor might be found.

The parents, devout Roman Catholics, wanted very much to have another child, especially a son. Within a month of the baby's death, Carol Ann conceived for the third time. The parents, Dr. Raphael Wilson (a gnotobiologist and Roman Catholic brother), and the two physicians, chose the technology of the germ-free environment. In the seventh month of pregnancy, amniocentesis indicated that Carol Ann carried a male child.

Five seconds after delivery by cesarean section on September 21, 1971, the baby was deposited in a sterile plastic isolator. David Phillip was baptized by his godfather, Raphael Wilson, with sterilized holy water that had been placed inside the bubble. He was immediately wheeled down the hall from St. Luke's Episcopal Hospital to a room in the Clinical Research Center (CRC) at adjoining Texas Children's Hospital (TCH). The infant appeared normal except for the absence of palpable lymph nodes. But an X-ray taken four hours after birth showed the absence of a thymus, the spongy gland normally located behind the breastbone. Specialized infection fighting white blood cells, known as T-cells, are produced in an immature form in bone marrow and grow to maturity in the thymus.

The second son had inherited the deadly gene. Two weeks later, after further tests, the doctors told the parents their second son had no immune system. A second isolator system was built for little David at his home and within two months he began to divide his time between his bubbles, at home and at the hospital.

Local newspaper reporters quickly learned of David's unusual birth but agreed to hold off on the story until the doctors had presented the case at a scientific meeting. On December 4, 1971, an article titled "Infant Tucked into Germ-Free World of Isolator—Hope to Overcome Usually Fatal Disease" appeared in the *Houston Chronicle*. Four days later, the *Houston Chronicle* quoted one doctor describing the team effort as "the most exciting drama" of his career. The story of the ten-week-old infant in an isolator caught the interest of the news media throughout the world. The cameras and journalists were welcomed. By the time he was one year of age, David's good looks and charisma had captured the imagination and fancy of the public. The news media gave David, the Bubble Baby, to the world.

2.

AGE THREE—THE HAPPY TIME

David is sick. He is dying. He has been removed from the bubble, and we are together in a sterile hospital room. He has extracted a promise from me to write this book, and we are discussing the details.

"I know exactly what you are going to say—you weren't around when it all started, you had nothing to do with anything till I was three—but you were here and you talked to all of them. You know everything."

"You're right on most counts. Actually the only person I ever discussed the original decision with was Raphael Wilson. He told me he had worked with the immune-deficient twins in Ulm, Germany. They were retarded, but so was the mother, and the father was in prison for the criminally insane. Your parents were intelligent and healthy, so for him that made you the perfect baby. He was always optimistic about a cure for you. Around the time your brother died, research breakthroughs in immunology looked promising. Many people thought that medicine would change—no more tooth decay, no more infectious diseases—but it wasn't that simple."

"Right. Look at the mess with AIDS. If those three had come up with some answers, they would have stayed here; you and Dr. Feigin wouldn't have been stuck with me."

"Don't include me in 'stuck.' My job was to test you and write a psychological report—that's all. I decided to work with you. At the time, it provided an exciting challenge and rare opportunity to study human development. Besides, I liked you; you liked me. I chose to love you."

"Call it love at first sight. I remember the first time we met."

"Silly—I doubt if you really remember. You repeated the story a hundred times when you were little, and you read my notes last summer when we were working on the perception paper."

"No, no, I remember. Let me tell you. A few days after my third birthday, you and another psychologist came to my house. He talked to my mother and you played with me. His car had the lights on because it was dark and pouring down rain. You had little cars and lots of things in suitcases. You wanted to turn off the noisy blowers. You didn't know it would fog up and deflate—you didn't know anything at all about bubbles."

"You taught me quickly. You recited the emergency procedure for transfer to a portable generator in case of a power failure—quite a feat for a three-year-old. I was accustomed to looking down at little kids, but you were up on a table; so when you stood, I had to look up at you. I didn't like that. You were so grown up, your vocabulary amazing."

"Tell me what I said about the pictures."

"Your inability to name common items like 'key' or 'bed' surprised me. You would change the subject to something more familiar, or say, 'David can't see anything.' You called a carrot a 'tree,' a cupcake a 'wastebasket, it sure is full,' and a multi-paned window 'nine TV sets stacked together.'

"You didn't know 'leaf' and insisted that a tree was a green circle on a brown rectangle, not leaves, branches, and a trunk. I suggested, 'When your sister comes home from school and the rain quits, you watch her take a leaf from the tree in the front yard.' You refused to give up your belief or stop asking questions."

"I know. Finally you said, 'Well, Katherine will probably be too small to reach it anyway,' and you went out in the storm yourself and dropped your umbrella when you broke off the branch. You and the leaves were wet. You put a leaf under the crib so I could look at it."

I, too, vividly remember the day we met. On September 25, 1974, Dr. H. Barry Molish, chief psychologist at TCH, and I drove forty miles to David's home in Conroe. Our evaluation was to be included in a case history of David in *The Journal of Pediatric Research*.

Although David's hospital room was just down the hall from my office in the Center for Developmental Pediatrics (CDP), I knew little about him, except what I had read in previous reports. At eight months, his language was delayed; he babbled while playing, but made no effort by sound or gesture to imitate or interact with familiar people. Rhythmic rocking came to occupy more and more of his time. A speech therapist taught the nurses to interact in ways to enhance his language and discouraged their perfunctory manner of carrying out duties. By the age of sixteen months, he had made great gains in language and continued to do so.

David's articulate but somewhat unusual speech, spontaneity, and effervescent personality intrigued me immediately. Also, he could not have been more beautiful: eyes deep, dark pools, blue-black hair, and olive skin. I had never encountered a child more eager to learn; to know.

His home life-support system seemed unreal, like something out of science fiction. The two isolators, made of twenty-mil polyvinylchloride (PVC), connected by an eighteen-inch diameter by eighteen-inch long sleeve, rested on tables in the living-and-dining area. David lived in what he referred to as the "crib," which was two feet by five feet by forty-two inches high. The other isolator, called the "supply," contained food, clothes, water, disposable diapers, washcloths, and trash bags. There were size nine men's neoprene gloves installed in the side of the crib to allow a caregiver to handle David—David could push the gloves inside out and theoretically use them to manipulate objects outside the bubble, but they were far too big to be really useful to him. Blowers, pumping sterile, filtered air inside the bubbles, made a constant whirring sound over which David and others had to speak in a near shout. As I played and worked with him, I couldn't help wondering how this precocious child could ever manage to survive in this confined space.

I noted disturbing behaviors. David never sat down. He either squatted or knelt with his bottom resting on his heels. If idle, he knelt, rocking and thumb sucking.

Further, he was surrounded by infant toys and drank from a bottle with a nipple. His mother referred to him as "Baby David."

It never occurred to me then that in ten days I would be seeing this child each day and that he would find a place for himself in my life.

David returned to the hospital on September 28, 1974, three days after my visit to his home. On October 7, Dr. John Montgomery, one of the original three doctors, thanked Dr. Murdina Desmond, my boss, for my having succeeded in testing David. He also discussed David's refusal to go into the Plexiglas playroom that had been built and connected to the hospital crib in March. Because Carol Ann had told him of my rapport with her son, he thought possibly I could persuade David to go into the playroom.

My days as a member of the multidisciplinary diagnostic team for children with problems were busy, busy. But since I seldom had appointments after four, I visited David late that same afternoon.

"*Lady!* You brought me the leaf. Katherine was too little; she couldn't get it; you had to get it. Where are your cars?"

He chattered on and on. He politely dismissed my suggestion that he go into the playroom. He objected to my leaving, looked me straight in the eyes, and stated, "Lady, you will be back. Bring me little cars."

Late the next afternoon, I stayed with him nearly two hours. He asked, "Lady, what's your name?" By now, we were friends.

At my request, he made several attempts to go into the playroom, but each time he stuck his head through the port, he cried, "It hurts my ears!" Because Plexiglas absorbs sound, an intercom system had been installed in the playroom to allow him to hear and be heard. It occurred to me the screeching intercom did, indeed, hurt his ears, and I had it turned off. But he still insisted, "It hurts." He steadfastly denied being afraid to go down the two-step ladder.

I promised to return and to buy him a little car for inside the bubble. "I want one that opens the doors, the front and the back," he ordered.

Not being prepared for David's aversion to the playroom, I questioned Ellen Hunt Hilton, a biologist and his primary caretaker. She said that on one of David's attempts to enter the new room, he had hit his head on the metal port.

Since cajoling did not entice him into the playroom, I made use of his good intelligence and eagerness to learn. I borrowed the goldfish that belonged to Mildred Carr, the CDP receptionist, and set the bowl on the floor by the far corner of the playroom. He zipped into the supply bubble to get a better view and asked me to hold it up, but I said, "I'm going to sit on the floor and watch the fish swim, you come over here."

As I had hoped, curiosity got the better of him; he had to investigate. He climbed down into the playroom so he could watch the fish. Three afternoons of watching a "real fish," and his fear of the playroom vanished.

Ellen, who had helped to construct the PVC bubbles before David was born, expressed her frustrations. So many people were involved in David's care that it was impossible to establish any order in his world. She asked for help in managing David's angry, hysterical outbursts and crying spells during which he dumped food and threw glass bottles. Even worse, he tore up disposable diapers, and the fuzz clogged the air outlets.

I questioned, "He's toilet trained, so why the diapers?" "We use them to line the potty," she said.

Kay Miller, the CRC administrator; Elaine Potts, the nutritionist, and several nurses voiced concern. It seemed clear to me that the major problem was that the nurses were accustomed to taking care of sick, compliant children, not an active, clever, robust three-year-old boy eager to assert his independence.

Reporting my success regarding the playroom stalemate to Dr. Desmond, I said, "The playroom problem is minor compared to the general chaos on CRC. No one is ready to deal with the prospect of Baby David growing up in the bubble. The nurses battle with him and with each other. The three-to-eleven shift and day shift barely speak. The evening nurses blame the day shift for potty spillovers. The day shift accuses the night shift of putting trash in with dirty clothes. Each believes the other shirks her lint picking duty. (Dozens of white washcloths went in the bubble, and each one had to be inspected for foreign particles and loose lint before it was sterilized.)

"David creates havoc by pitting the nurses against each other. He eats and sleeps when he pleases. He's bored and he's alone too much. He has no structured activities, no privacy, and no way to reach toys on the outside. This boy lives in a completely bounded world, yet in his world there are no boundaries."

"They need a team approach," Dr. Desmond responded. "Social work, play therapy, physical therapy, and psychology." She made it clear that David's psychological development would be up to Dr. Molish and me. With Dr. Montgomery's blessing, Dr. Desmond took charge and created the developmental support team from the multidisciplinary professionals in the Center for Developmental Pediatrics. We became the CDP team.

I soon learned about the important players in the convoluted drama, and how David's predicament elicited intense emotions and affected people's behavior. Some reacted with compassion and loyalty; others, revolted, could not tolerate being near him. A few considered him an oddity to be stared at or tormented, as a cruel child might tease a helpless animal in a cage. Many professionals let their respect for a human being go down the drain when working with David.

No wonder David mastered manipulation; he learned from the experts. He either liked or disliked a person, no in-between. To his friends, he was loyal and never betrayed a confidence. Carol Ann correctly stated, "My son plays a different role for each one he loves, the role he knows they want."

While it would be natural to suppose that his mother, Carol Ann, had the lead role in David's life, that was not always the case. Always beautiful, always impeccably groomed, proper, the perfect hostess, it was not in her nature to tell doctors and nurses what to do. Originally, I found her tendency to withdraw from conflicts—and sometimes from David himself—annoying, but as the years passed, I grew to admire her greatly. Faced with what was clearly an intolerable situation, I feel she handled it better than most people could have.

Her husband, David Sr., was what I would describe as a "typical Texan." Though he worked as a certified public accountant, he looked more like a rancher: he always wore cowboy boots, had a gun rack in his pickup truck, loved to hunt, fish, and drink beer. He was, I later found, a man capable of deep caring, but he found it difficult to relate to his son through the walls of the bubble. Like Carol Ann, he also tended to defer to the doctors' wishes.

While neither of David's parents enjoyed the limelight, Dr. Raphael Wilson loved it. A gnotobiologist (an expert in germ-free environments), a brother in the Holy Cross Order, and David's godfather, he ran the show. Prior to David's birth, he counseled the parents, advised on the sterile delivery, and designed the germ-free isolator. He had had previous experience with infants in a germ-free environment—twins in Germany and a child in Alabama. I thought of suave, articulate Raphael as "cerebral."

Raphael took enormous pride in his project—the isolator and David's brilliance. Despite his ostentatious publicizing of the Bubble Boy, he cared for David and spent a great deal of time with him. David enjoyed his company and emulated his speech and mannerisms. He said, "Dr. Wilson and I have man-to-man talks."

Ellen Hilton worked directly for Dr. Wilson. Her job of maintaining the germ-free environment was hard, tedious, time-consuming, and meticulous labor. Originally, she had been told her duties as a technician did not include spending time relating to David. However, when she discovered that he was often lonely and unhappy, she spent many work hours in his room so he would not be alone. He enjoyed watching her load cylinders and construct or repair bubbles. He depended on her for company and survival.

Elaine Potts made a career of David's nutrition. She supervised the culturing process and searched for germ-free food. Few foods could pass the rigid quality-control test; for the most part, he ate baby food. Potts and David dearly loved each other. She tried to make his life more pleasant by providing extras—bright balloons, holiday decorations, clothes, toys, and presents for David to give to his mother. He worried about her worrying about him. When her mother died, he mourned, not because he felt a loss, but because "Potts is so sad, I can't bear to think of how sad she feels."

Two nurses were important in David's life, Dorothy Johnson and Elizabeth Pollard. Both were dignified, competent, practical women who always seemed able to rise above the bickering. They maintained a rather distant, professional stance with David, but they cared. Elizabeth confided, "One winter morning when he was two, I woke him up at one in the morning to watch it snow. I was afraid he might never see snow. The next day, everyone questioned David: 'Why did you sleep till noon?' He never told."

But not all of David's nurses were so sympathetic. Some were cruel and so resented David that they taunted him—one would set him up to get into trouble with another. Others vied for his love, wanting to be the Bubble Boy's favorite.

They all seemed to agree on just one thing: their anger toward "Aunt Patty."

"Who is Aunt Patty?" I asked Ellen.

"Patricia Bealmear, a former nun and David's godmother." "David says she visits every night and has baby mice."

"Like Dr. Wilson, she has a doctorate in Gnotobiology from Notre Dame," Ellen explained. "She runs rats in germ-free isolators similar to David's system."

"Why is everyone angry?"

"Because Dr. Bealmear believes David belongs to her. She doesn't speak to Dr. Wilson and she's on the outs with Carol Ann. Miss Potts battles with her over the baby bottles, and she scares the nurses."

In person, Aunt Patty struck me as bigger and more overwhelming than her reputation. Within five minutes I knew her opinion on everyone concerned with David. She explained her labors to establish a strain of rats with an immune system identical to David's. A rat model could, perhaps, lead to a cure. (She kept me posted on her progress; later, a careless technician ruined her years of work.)

She lambasted the physicians for not attempting a fetal thymus transplant in David's first year of life. She firmly believed that for a transplant to be effective in reconstituting the immune system, it had to be done as near to the organism's fetal state as possible. Now, for David at three years, it was too late. Aunt Patty told me she started spending evenings with David when he was nine months old. "He was pathetic, so alone. Someone had to be with him."

Aunt Patty helped Ellen and the nurses. She prepared supplies, sterilized items, removed trash, and took care of David from six in the evening until he fell asleep. Conflicts arose with the staff and with Carol Ann as Aunt Patty became more and more possessive of David. She had been wonderful with and for him when he had been an infant and toddler—she taught him to count and to recite the alphabet and prayers—but seemed unable to accept his growing up. At age three, he resisted her authority, and his attempts at independence provoked battles.

After Raphael and Ellen indoctrinated me as to how they maintained the gnotobiotic state, I realized that David's confinement to a small space was the least of his deprivation. Everything he ate or touched, as well as the very air he breathed, had to be germ-free. Items inside the bubble had to be kept perfectly clean and dry—no urine drips, no spills.

The restrictions on what could go into the isolator eliminated virtually everything a little boy needed: nothing porous or painted, no wood, glue, or oil. I soon learned that almost everything had lubricants—a telescope, a doll's face, and most toys. Cloth, paper, smooth polished metals, glass, and many plastics could go in the isolator, but the sterilization process caused problems—holes had to be punched in hollow plastic toys in order to kill any germs that lurked in the interior. A punctured ball does not bounce, it plops. What good is paper if you can't have pencils, crayons, or glue?

David couldn't play effectively with anything outside the bubble because he had to stick his arm into a plastic sleeve that terminated in a huge, man's glove. He became quite adept at working in the big glove, although it seemed to me he might as well have put his hand in a man's wading boot.

The main, or "crib," isolator was attached to the "supply" isolator, which was also about ten square feet, by an eighteen-inch-diameter "sleeve." The crib isolator was the only one of the two isolators in which David could stand. The bubbles also had eighteen-inch-diameter "ports" that functioned as doors and were used to put in supplies and take out trash.

Everything David ate, wore, or came in contact with was packed in twelve-inch-diameter metal cylinders of three sizes, up to twenty-four inches long. The open end of a packed cylinder was closed with Mylar film and tape. The large cylinders were sterilized at the neighboring Methodist Hospital with ethylene oxide gas at 140 degrees Fahrenheit for four hours and room-aerated for seven days. Small cylinders were gassed in St. Luke's Hospital for ninety minutes and then put in an aerator for eight hours. Some items were autoclaved (bathed in 270 degrees Fahrenheit steam for thirty minutes).

Putting the supplies into the isolator was time consuming, hard, physical work. Cylinders were connected to the supply porthole by a tapered PVC sleeve after untaping the outside cap on the port. The connecting sleeve was taped to both the port and cylinder by yards and yards of fiberglass and vinyl tape. No creases or wrinkles were allowed. Aerosol two percent peracetic acid was sprayed through a plug in the airlock formed by the sealed sleeve. After a twenty-minute wait, the inner cap (held by two rubber bands which were three-fourths-inch wide) was taken off and the cylinder pushed to the port by compressing the sleeve accordion-style. Then the Mylar was popped from the inside and supplies unloaded. Trash was stuffed in the empty cylinder, and the inside bubble cap replaced before the sleeve was untaped. After taping the outside cap back, acid was sprayed in the airlock between the caps. Peracetic acid does not sterilize through particles; therefore, everything had to be absolutely free of dust, lint, and fingerprints.

Plastic containers with sterile contents bypassed the cylinder process and were put directly in the port and acid-sprayed, a forty-minute process.

In short, supplying David allowed for no spontaneity and little variety. Giving anything to him was complex. On October 8, 1974, I promised him a little car. On January 27, 1975, the first item on the packing list revealed the goal was nearing: Mary, dump truck (actually a tow truck) with a working pulley, VW, and sports car. Two weeks later he had the cars inside.

"What are you thinking about?" David asked.

"I'm remembering our beginning, how we played, how we had fun, and those rhymes you made up—Tickle, tickle, Doctor Nichols; Darling Dr. Starling; Watermelon, melon, Ellen; Hotsy totsy, here comes Potsy."

"Three was the happy time. I didn't care about problems. If I had one, it was fixed when you walked in the door. When I was three you could fix anything. When I got older, the problems got bigger, and you didn't have the power to fix them—no one did. If anyone could, it was you. Remember playing cars and bringing car pictures?"

"Those advertising pamphlets came from car dealers. I needed help to answer your questions. Cars never interested me—still don't, I learned more about cars than I ever cared to know. You had strange ideas, you called the hood the front door, the trunk the back door, and you insisted the back window was a windshield. You liked the little sports car I gave you because it had 'two chairs.'"

"We counted cars on Fannin Street by color, make, model, size. I watched you read and write down the names of the cars in the parking lot. You made me an expert on engines, brakes, transmissions, everything. I'll tell you something, I still don't understand why the rear window isn't a windshield!" We both laughed.

"When you were three, I was foolish enough to think I could teach you anything."

"You should have kept the pretty green LTD and not drove your son's ugly white Datsun 280Z. Your silver Mustang is pretty; still, you shouldn't have sold that Ford."

"You were five when I sold it. You ordered, 'Go get it back!' and cried when I said I couldn't."

"Selling that car was a mistake. By the way, where are you parking now that I am out and in this room?"

Such egocentricity. The world revolves around him; he comes out of the bubble and moves across the hall; therefore, I change my parking.

"The same place," I told him.

"Well, I guess you can't break a habit."

David and I had fun; however, no one but he would describe his third year as "the happy time." My visits with him and management tips to Ellen were just a drop in the bucket. It took the force of Dr. Desmond, a full Baylor professor with a formidable reputation, and the expertise of the CDP team to make progress.

On December 8, 1974, Dr. Desmond, Louise Haine (a social worker), Joan Sheldon (a child developmentalist), and I started planning our strategy to straighten out David's world.

The major problem centered around mealtimes: he preferred baby bottles of Enfamil formula and had little interest in other food. Accordingly, the nurses treated him like a baby, yet they demanded he act like an adult. He dare not drop one bite of food, any mess had to be immediately cleaned up, or bacteria, fungi, or spores would grow. If left alone, he dawdled or played in his food, making a mess.

Each morning, he decided which nurse he liked the best and only she would be allowed to "open" his food.

Right before Christmas, one nurse caught him dumping food in the trash bag and spanked him. He became hysterical, and they had a terrible time getting him settled down. Appalled at learning of the spankings, I explained that spankings merely intensified his oppositional behavior. No one heeded my objection, in part because his mother gave permission—she believed in discipline. Before he learned to scamper into the playroom and out of reach, it was easy to catch and spank him in the crib.

On January 15, 1975, Dr. Desmond chaired the first of many "CDP meetings" with Aunt Patty conspicuously absent. Establishing a schedule took priority: meals, bed, and bath (a wipe down with a damp washcloth) at regular times. Joan made lesson plans to be carried out by her and the CRC staff. Naively, Dr. Desmond believed her directive of gradually taking away nipples and her proclamation, "David is a preschooler," would end the crisis.

But it took more than a schedule and a doctor's orders to eliminate the nurses' bickering and rivalry. Today one nurse would be David's favorite, tomorrow another; he decided who did what: He fought to hold onto his control and had a staunch ally in Aunt Patty, who adamantly opposed the schedule. She liked the idea of his having a nap at four in the afternoon and staying up late with her. As she put it, "Baby David should have baby bottles."

As a part of Joan's first lesson plan of body awareness, a full-length mirror was mounted on a wall of the playroom. David became quite vain about his appearance. He noticed his black teeth and was eager to let a dentist clean them. We were afraid his teeth were decaying since Aunt Patty's germ-free rats' teeth also turned black. But the "black" chipped off, and the lab found it to be iron from the Enfamil. David ate no roughage to scour his teeth. His vanity kept him "brushing" daily with sterilized pumice and cooperating with frequent dental cleanings.

The following week, Louise started group therapy with the CRC staff and nurses. The day shift stayed late and the evening shift came early. The enormously popular sessions allowed everyone to vent feelings and gain insight. A nurse was "assigned" to David each day, an indirect way to limit his manipulations. Behavior management was addressed and spanking discouraged. The tension diminished.

Still, Dr. Desmond's directives did not produce a turnaround in the nipple battle, so she wrote specific orders in David's medical chart as to how they were to be gradually taken away.

When Aunt Patty read the order, she charged down to Louise's office, denounced her, and then confronted me. We thought a giant steamroller had smashed us flat. Louise reasoned, "Neither one of us is a match for her. From now on, we face her together, not singly." The next time she confronted us, we remained standing in the hall and held our position. It wasn't easy; She hadn't been on speaking terms with David's mother but now enlisted her aid to resist CDP's plans. Carol Ann, finally worn down, told Louise, "Whatever Aunt Patty says about the bottles is fine with me."

The battle of the nipples went on for six months. David hid them and the nurses' search accelerated, but he always had one. The little disposable bottles of Enfamil continued to be his source of milk. If he had a nipple, he could screw it on the bottle. He blamed or gave me credit for the nipple order and defied me, taunting, "You'll never find all the nipples. I will always have one—Aunt Patty will spray one in." At least he didn't have a nipple anytime he wanted. Sneaking around about it became a game, being one step ahead of everybody became as important as the nipple itself.

But always, David greeted me with a big smile and excitement—he was so open in expressing delight at seeing and being with me. His happiness was contagious. He shared his antics with me and asked thousands of questions. "Who gives you food? Do you have a daddy? Do you have a window?"

Laughing, he told me about his "bath." Ellen had taken everything out of the crib, sprayed in bottle after bottle of water, and poured the water into the crib. It was about time; David and the bubble both needed a good cleaning. He said, "I made a big splash and watched the water wiggle. Boy, I made a big mess with the water."

3.

AGE FOUR—DAVID MEETS FRIEND NUMBER TWO

"They should have taken me out when I was three. It would have been easier then—I'd be too young to know or care what was happening. Right?"

"Love, I don't know. I suppose you are partly right." "I didn't expect you to answer—no one has answers."

My thoughts drifted back to the beautiful, healthy little boy—exuberant and smiling.

At age three, he adhered slavishly to the tyranny of remaining germ-free. Nothing made me more furious than to hear professionals refer to David's "germ phobia." His fear was not irrational; every day, from day one, the danger of germs was pounded into him. He sought to dodge germs the way a soldier dodges bullets on a battlefield. Although he was knowledgeable about germs, he also had magical beliefs; for example, that a germ was a ferocious, attacking shark.

I marveled as the little tyke explained his ventilation system: "The blowers inflate the bubble and positive air pressure keeps germs from coming in a tear. Bacteria can't get through the spun glass in the filters, and tiny viruses always stick to a particle of dust so they get trapped, too. The outlets have filters, two, just in case air backs up."

Raphael confided, "The system is not foolproof. I never expected it to operate this many years without a major problem."

The hospital, Baylor, and NASA routinely monitored for microorganisms. David did not remain germ-free; by age two, eighteen different organisms had been isolated from his feces, urine, skin, or saliva. Many disappeared spontaneously, antibiotics eliminated some, and others colonized harmlessly in his gastrointestinal tract, but were potentially fatal if released in his bloodstream. The goal, then, became to maintain him in a disease-free, rather than a germ-free state.

Surveillance for cracks, pinholes, and weak spots in the bubble skin and the gloves was constant. David was quick to caution, "Take your rings and wristwatch off before you go in the gloves. Don't lean against the bubble—your buttons might be sharp!" He didn't dare be boisterous.

Yet, as a toddler, he was inconsistent. He once took a metal spoon and aimlessly hit the handle on the connecting sleeve, making a hole. Hospital staffers reprimanded him and demanded he explain his action. What three-year-old could tell you why he banged a spoon?

I pushed for small gloves. To my disbelief, child-size gloves could not be considered because the porcelain mold would cost fifty thousand dollars. A less precise mold would produce a glove with imperfections or weak spots. A man's .25-mil neoprene glove, although perfect, cost only twenty-nine dollars because of mass production for laboratories. I suggested small women's gloves, but if they existed they were never found. It was not until David was seven that he had both a right and left fitted glove, and a whole new world opened for him.

I also pushed for privacy, and my struggle here was more difficult. Even Potts was against installing curtains. "David has to be in full view at all times. What if he stopped breathing?" she asked.

David's hospital bubbles were in two hospital rooms, with most of the dividing wall removed. The supply bubble was about twelve square feet, but was generally so packed with food, linens, medical supplies, and so forth that David could only poke his head into it. The crib bubble, which sat on a tabletop, was about eighteen square feet, and the Plexiglas walled playroom bubble about forty-eight square feet. In other words, David's whole world in the hospital was confined to seventy square feet—and the bubbles that were constructed at his home once he grew past the toddler stage were about the same size.

In the hospital, one could not walk completely around the system. To get between the window and crib, you had twelve inches to squeeze through. David always reminded me, "You can't gain weight, and you won't make it."

Because of the two wide doorways, David was on display to anyone who strolled down the hall. David said, "They stretch their necks." He hated "gooseneckers" and often acted silly for them. At age five he said, "If they want to see a monkey in a cage, I'll be one."

Along with attracting the casually curious, David was a stop on the VIP tour. Opera star Beverly Sills, a European princess, and an Asian prince all came to gawk. Entourages of residents, students, and chaplains came in and treated David like a medical sideshow: "This is the boy with the X-linked combined immune deficiency, whose older brother...."

In March 1975, Dr. Desmond succeeded in getting the administration to distribute the first of many letters limiting visitors. Signs were posted, but many physicians did not believe the restriction applied to them.

David had no inhibitions; toileting was, for him, no different from taking a drink of water. No matter what or who, down went the pants.

I told him, "Pottying is private—when you have to go, say turn your back." He laughed, but agreed, and eventually made sure to ask all present to turn their backs whenever he used his toilet.

Finally, Dr. George Clayton, the director of CRC, agreed to cut a doorway between the adjoining storage room and David's quarters. Coming in from the storage room, one came face to face with the end of the supply isolator, and the TV was to the left. When David was in the crib and the hall door was closed, one could not see him from the hall. At least he had some degree of privacy. Still, I wanted curtains for the three Plexiglas walls of the playroom and another across the hall door. Five years later, red—David's choice—drapes were installed inside the playroom.

Carol Ann attended several CDP meetings and talked with Louise a couple of times. After their first session Louise recognized two major problems: Carol Ann had never had time to grieve for the first "Baby David," and the hospital had "usurped" the parents' role or Carol Ann and David Sr. had relinquished responsibility. Louise's goals were to counsel Carol Ann and to help both parents take an active role in decision making.

David Sr. declined to participate in meetings. A caring, private man, he had made the tables for the bubbles.

Much to David's delight, he once stayed all night at the hospital. The next day David complained, "Potsy, the girls didn't feed my Dad!"

Carol Ann's weekday CRC visits were gourmet tea parties with the lavish pastries she made for the staff. She, with David's father and sister, usually visited on Sunday afternoon.

Louise contacted the Conroe Independent School District to have David classified as handicapped and, therefore, eligible for an early childhood education program. Arden Richardson, head of special education, became David's advocate, and through her efforts, which offended the physicians, the parents, and the hospital attorney, his schooling approached normalcy. In August 1975, the teacher started coming to the hospital and his home two times per week.

When I first met David, my life was complicated by the illness of my brother's wife. She remained in The Methodist Hospital from September 1974 until her death in July 1975. My five-year-old niece, Renee, often accompanied me visiting David late in the afternoon. After we left him, we walked the short distance to The Methodist Hospital to see her mother.

On Renee's first visit, David shouted, "Get out! Don't touch that, it's mine!"

She dealt effectively with three older brothers, so his verbal assaults and orders didn't intimidate her. She placed her fists on her waist, looked him straight in the eye and demanded, "Do you want me to stay or go? Make up your mind!"

He yielded. "Stay."

I enjoyed being with these two bright, vivacious children. David considered Renee beautiful. His incessant questions did not annoy her, even though many were about her mother. She told him, "My mother is going to die but it's all right—she will be beautiful again and not hurt anymore."

After her death, David said, "Well, I hear your mother finally died. Did you cry? Were you sad?" The nurse, in tears, signaled no.

I interrupted, "Let them talk." Death, real or potential, was a looming reality in the lives of both these young children, and it seemed appropriate to allow them to air their questions and feelings about it. Soon they were playing, the conversation ended.

Renee became infatuated with a scraggly-legged, green plush frog with a white tummy that lay on the window ledge. As she cuddled it, David demanded, "Put it down. That's my frog!"

"You don't care about that frog," I admonished him. "You've never paid any attention to it. Let her play with it." Miffed, he relented.

As we were leaving, she asked him for it. "No! It's mine! I love it!" he shouted.

She cried. Then he cried, because I requested he lend her the frog. As he tearfully refused, I consoled Renee by saying he'd change his mind.

On my next visit I asked, "Where is the frog?"

"It's on its way to Methodist." In other words, it was being sterilized. A week later, the frog, minus its glued-on eyes, entered the bubble. As he tightly hugged it, his defiant expression conveyed, "She'll never get it now!"

But later that same evening, he came to realize how insignificant his victory was compared to the enormity of his isolation. True enough, Renee did not have the frog, "But she gets to go every place with you."

In the early months of 1975, when he was three, David's world expanded beyond the lesson plans: The TCH Women's Auxiliary replaced his twelve-inch black-and-white TV with a nineteen-inch color set. On March 3, Tom Langford, head of electrical services, installed it.

Before it was turned on, David seemed disappointed. "I thought it was going to be a color TV—a red one." But when it was switched on, he understood. "Oh, it's lots of colors! Mr. Langford, I sure do thank you."

Mr. Langford, one of David's favorite people and one of the few he trusted, personally supervised all of the electrical work on the isolator. He enjoyed Tom's visits and equipment inspections at the hospital and at his house.

Aunt Patty brought mice. David saw her coming, bearing a blue package, and yelled to the nurse, "You'd better leave or you'll get really scared. I think they're mice!" He squashed and killed one trying to hold it with the big glove.

Later, he told me he had actually held them inside the bubble: "Aunt Patty sprayed in pink babies for me to play with." It may have been true, since it was possible and she had expressed the desire to do so. Her germ-free mice could have been put in a sterile container and sprayed into David's bubble. After all, she knew he wouldn't tell.

"Touching something warm and alive might diminish his thumb sucking and rocking," she'd reasoned.

To expand David's world beyond his hospital and home isolators, Raphael set the supply bubble on a patient gurney and took David on a tour. In the twenty minutes he could remain disconnected, he wanted to see Potsy's kitchen, go through the swinging doors to the maternity ward, and to my office. What astonishment to see a flushing toilet and so many babies! He was bouncing around, laughing and counting doors when we hit a snag—the bubble's baseboard was too wide to go through the CDP door, so he could not see my office.

Unfortunately, the door was near an outside entrance. People surrounded us, shouting, "It's the Bubble Baby!" "Look!" "He's so cute!" "He looks just like his pictures!"

Startled and frightened, David scrunched up in a ball; lips quivering and eyes huge, he stuffed his hand in his mouth. Ignoring my protest, a woman poked the bubble. I pushed her aside and stood between her and the bubble. Oblivious to our frantic pleas and shouts to get away, the crowd thrust forward. I tried to shove people away as Raphael quickly rolled the bubble back to the elevator.

David looked relieved as we entered his room. "That's my bubble. I sure am glad I got to do this—I liked the babies. What did those people want? Why did that woman yell?" He then turned his attention to overseeing the reconnection.

I went to my office and cried. I couldn't get the look of terror in his eyes out of my mind. For the first time I had faced the morbid and potentially dangerous curiosity of the public. Seeing this child treated as a freak in a carnival side show hurt.

Also, I suddenly realized how much he meant to me, how much I cared, and what hurdles might await. Years later, David said, "You always move to protect me."

Louise's therapy sessions continued to go well until March, when she perceived something askew—a vague unease among the women in the group. She read the note of March 13, 1975, in David's chart and realized what was wrong—Dr. Montgomery was leaving for Alabama, and Dr. Buford Nichols was assuming charge. Although the nurses had been unaware of Dr. Montgomery's departure, they had sensed his "pulling out."

Devastated at learning of Montgomery's "desertion," David's mother came to Louise's office. It was, to her, the end of the world. "What will happen to David? Dr. Nichols isn't an immunologist." The team's and caretakers' reactions were almost as dramatic as Carol Ann's. Montgomery's departure ended the hope of a "cure" and talk of "when he comes out," making everyone more determined to hold on to the "baby." (Despite Dr. Desmond's all-out efforts, it took another two years before staffers stopped referring to David as a baby. The family, Dr. South, and the press, held on to "Baby David" even longer. His confinement and utter dependence upon others tended to cancel out the obvious fact that he was a bright little boy, not an infant.)

I was less than enthusiastic about Dr. Nichols's "temporary" tenure as David's primary physician. I had tested children for his research projects and considered him self-serving. Sure enough, the group therapy sessions ended quickly after he took over. As Louise put it, "He stood in the door and glared. No one would talk, and they eventually quit coming."

After attending several meetings, Dr. Barry Molish told me: "I give up. It's a hot potato—a political football. No one wants my input. I'll be useless to David all encumbered in the rivalry and battle for control. Everyone is invested and wants a part of the action, but no one is willing to actually get involved with the boy. You made your place with him. The powers are willing to give you a role because they don't want to put in any time or effort. You (he put his finger on my chest) stay. I can best help David by helping you. The affection between you two will keep you in there. I'll be here for you." He always was.

David didn't carry out his worst threat of smearing "poo-poo" all over the bubble and, except for his receiving and hiding Aunt Patty's contraband nipples, he adjusted well to the new regime. Much to the frustration of Potts, Aunt Patty continued to douse his nipples with acid. Potts equated this shortcut sterilization with poisoning.

Formidable as she was, Aunt Patty proved to be no match for Nichols. On May 15, 1975, he had a lock installed on the room housing the gas tank and acid. Within a few weeks, the last of the hidden cache of nipples was confiscated. Two Plexiglas boxes with combination locks, one for medical supplies and the other for food, were put in the supply. David could no longer ransack. Order was being established.

With the schedule well in place and the milk consumption curtailed, David still had no appetite. He told Potsy, "I want some big people's food—a bag of popcorn." The agenda for every CDP meeting included figuring out how to get him to eat. One morning when he was nine years old, the immunologist and I were with him while he ate his tepid, colorless, textureless, and probably tasteless, baby food breakfast. As we left, the doctor shook his head. "No wonder he doesn't eat!"

Potts struggled to balance and vary David's diet, even experimenting with baking in nylon bags. Her dream for him was a hamburger, French fries, and a Coke. Nothing worked. Fats and egg yolks never tested germ-free. His all-time favorite was chocolate pudding.

In later years, he had more variety, but he hesitated trying a new food and often waited for me to be present. Once, he screamed and keeled over with a piece of baked apple skin in his mouth. He had never before experienced texture in food.

Because little could be done to improve the food itself, Potts, Louise, and I labored to make mealtimes a pleasant social event. Raphael often joined David for lunch, and naturally David ate better on those occasions.

Now that he was no longer a compliant baby, David's relationship with Aunt Patty began to deteriorate. They quarreled, and to her horror, he began to say "damn" and "hell" instead of "Oh, for a child's grace."

David told a nurse, "I wore you out yesterday, didn't I?" He had fought hard against a needle being inserted in his arm; now, drawing blood was impossible until technicians rigged up a papoose board on which he was restrained with straps.

At three-and-a-half years, David had some awareness of his predicament and how his reactions affected the caretakers. He threatened, "I'll just get out and leave!"

He frequently pointed out that he wanted "to stay at home the rest of my life." He usually spent two to four weeks at home and then four at the hospital.

When he was four, things started going downhill even more rapidly. David returned to the hospital on January 11, 1976, for a month's stay and was labeled "a holy terror." He cried for no apparent reason and woke up screaming for "Mommy."

I read *The Monster at the End of This Book* to him a thousand times, but, otherwise, I failed in my attempts to interest David in books. His reaction frustrated me because I wanted him to know the pleasure of books. Sometimes, just to please me, he would let me read to him.

I felt his responses to pictures reflected not only his limited experience but also a desire to be a part of a family. His reaction to seeing a picture of a child in a crib: "The little boy is trying to tell his mother where he can go. He wants to go somewhere. He might walk out of that cage and go to church or some other building. Then he will come back and eat supper and go to bed and then keep on doing the same thing every day. He wants to play with neighbors." His reaction to seeing a picture of a man and a boy in a forest: "That man is crying because he can't get his son because he went far, far away to a neighbor's house. He'll go and try to straighten the little boy out."

I purchased a navel orange and white wristwatch while on a Caribbean cruise. David promptly noticed, admired, and longed for it.

"Where did you get that watch?" he asked. "I bought it on the ship."

"Oh, come on, you can't buy a watch on a ship. Where did you get it?" "Truly, I bought it in the gift shop on the ship."

"Oh, you just sit on a ship."

"The ship had a dining room, cabins, a swimming pool, and a theater. It was as long as the parking lot."

"No, no. The parking lot is the biggest thing in the whole world."

"We did not sit in a little rowboat on the ocean for two weeks—we were on a luxury liner with hundreds of people."

I'm not sure if this penetrated. After a long pause he said, "I sure do wish I could wear that watch." Had there been any way to sterilize the watch, I would have given it to him gladly.

Despite my years of efforts and demonstrations, he never grasped the concept of a body of water. My niece Renee once proudly told him how I had taught her to swim and to dive for pennies in my pool. He looked at her in bewilderment and said, "Let's talk about Mary's doggies, Bunchy and Susie."

"But Bunchy died, and Susie lives with grandmother," argued Renee. "Oh, oh, oh! Poor Mary, two dead daddies and a dead dog." He had successfully ended the "water" talk.

I tried balancing on a stool pretending to swim. I sailed paper boats in a pan of water. I sank objects, drew pictures, all to no avail. Sometimes his generalizations or perceptions exasperated me: On TV a boy running in a wheat field was "a boy swimming in the grass."

I had told Raphael that David didn't understand water. I simply couldn't teach him concepts having to do with space, depth, or distance. "Ridiculous," Raphael had said, "He's a bright boy." But later, he phoned, "I want to apologize. You were right. David didn't comprehend the account of my fishing trip. I tried several approaches. We will work on this when we get the space suit."

Dr. Nichols soon clashed with NASA officials who felt they had done more than their share in helping us with David. Also, his demands jeopardized other collaborative projects. Raphael tried to smooth things over and summed it up, "Without help from NASA we will be in severe straits indeed." I saw my pet project of getting a pencil in the bubble going down the drain. The Space and Life Sciences Directorate at NASA had one of the most sophisticated biological laboratories in the country. David's life would have been total deprivation without their expertise, facility and compassion. They tried anything we asked—if they couldn't do it, it couldn't be done. NASA, appeased by Baylor officials, continued the collaborative projects and to help David.

In the spring of 1976, everything changed for David. Three important people in his life—Ellen, Raphael, and Aunt Patty—quit their jobs. Ellen left at the end of March, the next week Raphael had a heart attack, and in May Aunt Patty moved to Buffalo, New York.

Ellen had found Nichols's contemptuous attitude and demands intolerable and, after much soul-searching and heartache at parting from the child she loved, she resigned. David mourned; so did his mother and I. Ellen visited often and continued to consult on his maintenance.

The weekend David learned that Raphael had had a massive coronary and was in intensive care at St. Luke's, he smeared "poo-poo" all over the bubble (requiring a three-day cleanup). Raphael recovered, but he went to the University of Oregon.

Aunt Patty's departure was, in part, precipitated by David's open warfare with her; he was trying to throw off her smothering love and control. To survive, she had to leave. She accepted an appointment with her former mentor. David went home on May 25, and she left the next day. Despite everything, she had filled a void in his life, and no one ever doubted her love for him. She was a true godmother.

Using the power of words, David lured the nurses into arguments and zinged them, hitting their weak spots. These behaviors would not have gotten out of hand if Louise's group sessions had been supported. Much to my distress, Louise left Baylor in May. Fortunately, she continued to be my advisor, friend, and confidante. The young man, Rock, who was trained by Ellen to take over, left after a few months.

Capable, officious Donna Curlin, R.N., became David's caretaker, but she did not successfully deal with David. "He tests my authority by using verbal contests to keep me in conflict with him," she complained. "Spankings don't work." She never sought my advice.

But David's tantrums ultimately began to wane. At Carol Ann's insistence, her son became more polite and respectful. Another reason for his increasingly compliant attitude was his growing awareness that he was utterly dependent upon those outside his bubble. He had an uncanny knack of rapidly assessing a person's motives, strengths, and weaknesses. He listened and watched for cues as to their interests and usually launched into a rapid inquiry, realizing, correctly, that people like to talk about themselves.

With all of this going for him as well as an excellent memory, unbelievable vocabulary, and quick wit, he developed poise and finesse in conversation. David perfected his publicly respectful stance and was so adroit at politely dismissing people that they seldom knew what happened: "It was so kind of you to visit, please do come back and let me know…."

Two very good things happened in the summer of 1976: the playroom at home was completed and Jackie Vogel, head of TCH Child Life/Play Therapy, joined the team.

Jackie worked with David daily during his hospital stays. After her first session, on July 16, 1976, his parting request was that she write the exact day and time of her return on his calendar. The little boy, who once knew no time boundaries or schedule now, at four-and-a-half years, functioned by clock and calendar.

His mastery of time concepts was precocious. Even though he didn't actually tell time, he used the clock: "Little hand at three and big hand at six—time for Jackie." Probably few, if any, other children ever gazed at a clock so much. Unable to go and get anything, he totally depended on people and things being delivered to his world, and lateness or changes in routine distressed him.

Jackie recounted her frustration and feeling of helplessness in trying to establish a relationship with David.

"It was very difficult. I had never before had difficulty getting to know a child, particularly a preschooler, because that's my favorite age group, my specialty. Usually I'm able to establish almost instant rapport with that age, even with kids who have the reputation of being difficult. So it was a real disappointment and puzzlement that it took so long to establish a relationship even though he was not hostile, or anything like that. It's just that it was very difficult to get to know him, and it was a long time before I felt he was comfortable with me.

"I think probably some of that was my being intimidated by the setup, the plastic, the gloves, by all the stuff that was in between us. It all had a certain mystique, plus it was a physical barrier. You couldn't always hear him as well as you wanted to; he couldn't hear you. So many of the activities that you would consider absolutely normal for that age group he couldn't take part in.

"He was always used to being very polite. It took a long time to know what was real and what he was saying because he knew that was what he was supposed to say. It took me a long time to figure out the difference between those two parts of him. That is, I guess, one of the things that kept me uncomfortable. I sensed he was being excruciatingly polite sometimes when he didn't really want to be. Most kids that ages don't have that kind of facade, they don't bother. If they don't want you, they slam the door, they let you know in some physical way that they're tired of participating. It was very hard for David to do that—he sensed his dependence on other people—he really didn't want to make you upset. He felt very vulnerable and was, therefore, much more polite and correct than what was called for in a four or five-year-old kid. I always felt that was a particular burden for him, but I never knew how to take it away, because it was so much a part of him."

From the beginning, Jackie and I had the best possible relationship. We had mutual respect and a similar philosophy about a child's needs. Without our ever discussing it, we presented a united front. Not once were we at odds, nor did we give differing advice.

Generally, David could not tolerate talking with more than one person. If two people faced each other rather than him, he could not follow the conversation because of the blowers' noise and the plastic's muffling effect. He did not like to share people, but he learned to enjoy Jackie and me together.

The mornings he left for home became a special sharing time. We waited for his mother to arrive—she followed the hospital van that carried David back to the house. We accompanied him to the basement garage and helped to lift the bubble into the van, which was equipped with a special power supply module to pump in fresh, filtered air. He was sad to leave his collective hospital mothers, but happy to go home to Mom, Dad, and Katherine. Home was where he belonged.

4.

HOW AND WHY

"It's settled, you'll leave for Singapore when this is over. Now, back to the subject you would rather not discuss. You've talked to the three doctors that started all this. You must have some idea what they were thinking. Why me? Why the research? Did they have second thoughts?"

"You've asked the same questions every day since you came out of the bubble. Dr. South and the other two gave you a chance to live. Thirteen years ago isolation seemed to be the answer. They thought you would be out and cured in three months." I thought back. Soon after we had met, I had attended a seminar, "Ethical Issues in Gnotobiology: The Case of Baby David." "No one had answers, just passionate, self-righteous opinions. It was so awful. I don't think I have ever discussed it with anyone."

On February 26, 1975, the Rev. Raymond J. Lawrence, director of Clinical Pastoral Education at St. Luke's/TCH, convened the conference on David with the cooperation and participation of Drs. Montgomery and Wilson. Mr. Lawrence invited Joseph Fletcher, Ph.D., a well-known professor of ethics at the University of Virginia Medical School, to speak.

At least thirty people crowded into the room; many stood against the walls. After the introduction, Raphael spoke. Supremely confident, he appeared to glory in occupying center stage. Rather than discuss the ethical dilemmas, he rather dryly recited David's case history, including a great deal of abstruse medical data, and concluded: "Research continues, not only for a cure for David, but also into the effects of isolation on his physical and psychological development. In the meantime, David gives every appearance of being a happy, well-adjusted, well-developed, and, occasionally, spoiled three-and-a-half-year-old...."

After that, all hell broke loose. Raphael's verbose, irrelevant digressions riled the group, which had convened with the intention of hashing out the ethical problems surrounding David's confinement.

Never in my life had I been a part of anything like this. It was unbelievable, the strong reactions David elicited in these people—hostility, repulsion, empathy, sorrow. Feelings, not reasoning, totally dominated. I sat there, stunned; keeping up with the verbal attacks and counterattacks were like trying to watch a tennis match.

Dr. Montgomery became defensive and angry when bombarded with questions he could or would not answer: "Is it right or wrong to make David a prisoner? Should there be a padlock on his isolator? Will you use "heroic psychological measures" when he resents being a guinea pig? Who pays? What is the benefit to society? What about when he's judicious enough to make his own decisions about sexuality, suicide, his humanness in years to come? What about real issues, family stress, caretakers' stress?

The exchange became most heated when Mr. Lawrence said, "My major concern, and my colleagues have expressed this same concern, is how will David negotiate puberty and handle his sexuality? In isolation he will have no sexual choices, no physical contact. My question is how, under these deprived conditions, can he remain human?"

Others passionately voiced similar views and feelings. This fiery discussion of sexuality further exacerbated the tension, the hostility, and some participants even began to cry. Apparently, the mention of sex, and the mere thought of a teenager confined to a bubble was more than these people could tolerate.

The discussion frequently touched upon suicide. At one point, an audience member pointed out that the decision to commit suicide is one faced by all severely handicapped, chronically ill people.

Dr. Fletcher said, "That is correct... I am going to Germany next month to read... my paper, 'In Defense of Suicide'... David might very well say, 'All right, you know, the flame is now no longer worth the candle.'"

The question of whether David was a boy or a research project had surfaced in other places. I had read the two original physicians' opinions in various publications. For example, quoting from an interview of Drs. Montgomery and South in *American Medical News,* November 21, 1977, long after they had left the project:

Dr. Montgomery: We never thought we would see him reach age six in isolation. We felt that in a year or so, at most, six months, the problem would be solved or he would have died. The question "What are we doing?" never occurred to me. We knew exactly from the start what we were doing. We would protect him by the best methods possible until we could find a bone marrow donor and the transplant would work. Or we would not find a donor, in which case we felt the isolation system would probably break down—and we would have done the best we could....

Would I do it again? Absolutely. If we had it all to do over again, would we go to the moon again...?

It has been a very successful investigational and therapeutic exercise and I see no reason to second-guess anything that we've done so far.

Dr. South: I thought [the first son's disease] was a new mutation, not a familial sort of case. We had no way of knowing whether the mother was indeed a carrier of the defective gene....

Dr. Montgomery: We knew more about SCID than genetics did at that time. We told them the probabilities. They asked what could be done if... only then did we tell them what was possible.

Dr. South: We did not conceive, it didn't even occur to anybody, that David would be in the protective environment this long. We didn't even really consider not to treat, but rather how to treat and would it be safe and useful to him, if it all became necessary.... I don't have one moment's regret. When I visit him and see him healthy and see him playing and laughing and absolutely normal developmentally in his growth and psychologically, I do not regret this all one bit. And he's happy, that's the main thing. Also, when I look at some forty papers people have written from his case, we've certainly gotten our money's worth. I've learned more immunology from him than just about anyone I can think of.

I hadn't known David very long when his dislike of Dr. Mary Ann South became apparent. I never heard him say her name; she was always *"she."* I assumed he associated her with blood drawing, but Ellen didn't think so. Years later, I recalled Ellen's speculative comment, "Maybe it's the skin graft.

It was painful. But I doubt that David would remember it—he was only five months old."

Ellen described the horrible fiasco. Dr. South wanted to graft another person's skin onto David; if he failed to reject it, it would be the ultimate proof of his immune deficiency. Ellen had become sick and almost fainted during the procedure, to which Dr. Wilson, out of character, had reacted, "If you can't take the heat, you better find another job!" Dr. South carefully explained to Carol Ann that the procedure would not benefit her son, but she needed the results for a scientific publication.

Dr. South, herself, donated the half-inch square of skin, which a plastic surgeon grafted onto David's left upper arm. To provide a comparison of any reaction, a patch of skin cut from David's own leg was grafted right next to hers. Any surgical procedure carries the risk of infection; the danger was compounded by the fact that, inadvertently, Aunt Patty and Ellen simultaneously took off the inside and outside caps and David was exposed to room air.

For the rest of his life, David resented the patch of fair skin, which resembled a white, burn-like scar. If anyone mentioned it, he shot a deadly, silent stare. The scar, for him, marred the perfection of his body of which he was so proud and, yet, at the same time, was a constant reminder of his imperfection.

David's feelings toward Dr. South caused him distress because his parents held her in the highest esteem and she was a frequent houseguest. Stomach aches became associated with her hospital visits. He would mumble, "I'm not her little boy." I met Dr. South several times, but she never spoke beyond a greeting.

David seldom mentioned Dr. Montgomery. The nurses liked this pleasant, dapper gentleman. Carol Ann had great faith in him as a physician and he provided her with emotional support.

Cloistered in this sterile, barren room, the colorless February days and nights did not differ The many necessary medical procedures meant little sleep at night, nor could we engage in any of the rituals we had established over the years: hide-and-go-seek, watching traffic on Fannin Street, or bumping foreheads hello and goodbye, as skin-to-skin contact was forbidden.

The TV, mounted high on the wall, provided some diversion. David watched the news bulletins on his condition. Erroneous details from past press conferences enraged him. "I never said I wanted to walk in the grass!

I never visited the parking lot! Some psychiatrist described how frightened I was coming out. Stupid! What does he know? He didn't even know you and Dr. Shearer were the only ones around! I'm telling you, when this is over, you tell the truth. Promise."

"Yes, I promise."

We reminisce, our eyes locked in silence: In our talks and in our minds we relive our lives together. David never forgot anything, probably because his memory wasn't cluttered with thousands of varied experiences and he never did or said anything just one time—stories were retold, events described again and again, and the same questions asked a hundred times. He repeatedly asked, "Remember when, remember when, remember when?"

I do remember.

5.

AGE FOUR—DAVID GAINS KNOWLEDGE

"Mary, don't you wish we had the record player in here with us? We could play our song. Remember the first time I played it for you?"

"Of course, love, how could I forget?"

At age nine, he had smiled and told me, "I have a special surprise for you. Listen." He had played Jim Henson as Kermit the Frog singing "The Rainbow Connection." After the words, "The dreamers and me," he had said, "That's you and me—the dreamers." Now, seeing tears in his eyes, I thought, Dreams can't stop death. I will drown in my own tears. How can we part? How can we ever say goodbye?

Jackie introduced the record player in the summer of 1976. It became an integral part of David's life. But it also became the source of a fair amount of trouble in what would prove to be a difficult year. David returned to the hospital on Monday, July 12, 1976, and, without Aunt Patty, reportedly cried all evening. Though intimidated by her, he had never before been without her at night. Tuesday afternoon his mood worried me so much that I went back to see him at half past seven. He was lying down sucking his thumb. "I miss Mommy, but she is coming Thursday," he said.

We played cars, exercised, and looked at a CRC scrapbook. Through the window he noticed that the 'H' light on top of the Shamrock Hilton was off and said, "We will have to call Aunt Patty and tell her to come to Houston and fix that 'H.'"

The next day his TV broke. Because it was privately owned, no one took the responsibility for repairing it. I called Mr. Langford. "Please...."

I spent the next four evenings with David, but his mood was sullen. He wouldn't do anything except play peek-a-boo or listen to any story except *The Monster at the End of This Book*. The effort to gain his interest and the frustration of not being able to engage him in varied activities wore me down.

My friend, Gary Whitney, an architect, offered to help. I knew David would object and consider Gary a rival for my attention. Sure enough, David reacted violently to Gary, shouting, "Get that man out of here!"

But patience won him over. The next evening, Gary brought a bowl of seashells and David had a new interest. I bought books on seashells, and soon David became quite an expert.

Gary, concerned about David's lack of privacy, had several ideas, including a "worm tunnel" or a tent, but none could be sterilized sufficiently to go in the bubble.

The next evening, when I walked in alone, it was clear Gary had won David over. "Where is Gary?" David demanded. "Why is he building a house in San Antonio? He should build one here!"

I visited every evening. Gary often accompanied me and played with David while I studied. Gary, determined to find a way for David to "get away from it all," told me to have extra receiving blankets put in the bubble so we could construct a tent.

"I told David how to drape the blankets over the table in the playroom, but each time he crawled in a blanket fell down. "Oh, I can't do it!" he cried.

"Oh, yes we can," I assured him. "Take a deep breath, settle down, and get some heavy things to set on top of the blankets. Before you crawl in, lift up the blanket so you don't pull it down."

"Finally in his tent, he stuck his head out, beaming. "I like it!" I did too. Every little boy needs a private hiding place, and David needed one desperately.

The CRC staff did not like his retreat. "What if something happened to him?" was a constant concern.

Annoyed, I contended, "What could possibly happen to him under there? Ye gads, the tent is right under a glove, you can yank it down in one second!"

Thursday, July 29, when I arrived, David was out of sorts—rocking, sucking his thumb, and generally irritable. He had had a fight with a nurse and refused to eat.

The pressure was mounting on him. Carol Ann had called and told him the family was coming in the next day to view the NASA "space suit" film.

The space suit was a germ-free, pressurized outfit that would allow David to leave his bubble and explore for short periods. Very important public relations people, engineers, and officials from NASA, Baylor, and the hospital would be there.

I tried to talk about the space suit. Distraught at the thought of being disconnected from the main system and taken to a room full of strangers, he whimpered, "I don't want to talk about tomorrow and the MBIS (Mobile Biological Isolation System)."

The next day, David's apprehension prevented him from absorbing anything from the film. I grew apprehensive, too; my illusions of freedom and action for him crumbled when I saw the complexity of the space suit. I knew it couldn't be simple, but I was surprised that it was tethered to a large, intimidating mobile apparatus by just an eight-foot hose.

In the film, a five-year-old girl modeling the suit was walking by a lake and swinging and seesawing at a playground.

"Did you have any problems getting the girl to go into the suit?" I asked the NASA personnel who had prepared the film. They replied that, indeed, the girl had been frightened and reluctant to get in. Just what I needed to hear!

Carol Ann brought a new record player on August 5. It was placed on the hospital table outside the bubble. The next week, the nurses complained about David's blank staring at the spinning, silent record player.

David went home on August 15 and returned six weeks later. His first day back, the nurses complained that he seemed to be hypnotizing himself with the record player, and he screamed if they turned it off. I was dumbfounded when I walked in and saw him on his knees in a zombie-like trance. Mesmerized, he moved like a charmed snake. All my attempts to engage him failed.

I knew it was crucial to extinguish this maladaptive, autistic behavior, so I told myself, "If you can't beat him, join him." I put a sheet of white paper over the spinning record and dripped on tempera paints. Focused on the turntable, he had no choice but to watch the paper and colors. Curiosity took over; he had to see what the paper looked like when the player was stopped. He then tried different colors and types of drips. From the psychedelic drawings, I moved to a tape recorder. We recorded his favorite record, thus eliminating the temptation to self-hypnotize when he was left alone.

After he had quit the self hypnosis and had begun to play appropriately, I intended to visit him occasionally, not every night. Upon learning this he wailed, "But you can't not come! What will I do? I can't go back!"

"Okay, I'll come tomorrow night." At that moment, without realizing all the implications, I voiced a commitment, a commitment I never broke.

By his fifth birthday, we had created what he referred to as "our private world." Behind closed doors, we shut out everything—the outside world ceased to exist. The ever present barrier of the PVC separated us physically, but never kept us apart. The isolator system, a noisy contraption, severely curtailed activities I wanted to initiate. Nevertheless, we engaged in the imaginative, sometimes boisterous play of children.

We worked out an agreement by which I would visit him every other night during his hospital stays—he generally spent four weeks at home, and four weeks at the hospital. Also, he charged, "Saturday nights are mine." I seldom, if ever, missed spending Saturday evening with him.

Then he bargained, successfully, for even more of my time. "Study here. I won't bother you. Your office is here and it's five minutes from school and the library." The month of his fifth birthday, he became intimately acquainted with the dedication necessary to achieve a doctorate.

Years later, David's first question on Jackie's announcement that she was going back to school was, "Will you have to do a research paper like Mary?" When she told him yes, he said, "Oh, oh my, Jackie, that's terrible! I've been through all that with Mary—it's awful. Now let me tell the problems. First, you have to get your committee together and then your subjects. Will you have a control group? How many? What about analysis?"

"I sat there with my mouth open," Jackie said. "I was thinking, I can't believe this—a nine-year-old laying out for me all the difficulties of getting a graduate degree."

Always, my focus was on allowing David to be a normal little boy, even when that was inconvenient for others.

For example, once Gary brought a box of sand with several hermit crabs in it. David soon lost interest in the crabs, but never in the sand. Fitted gloves would have allowed him to build sand castles, but stuck as he was with large gloves, he had a more devilish idea.

"Mary, I bet we could make a real mess with this sand."

"Okay, a mess you'll make. First let me spread a sheet over the motors. Then go at it."

He threw sand as best he could with the big gloves, and I scooped it up for him to throw again. Ecstatic, he wore himself out. We both laughed until we almost cried. It took me an hour to retrieve all the grains of sand; he supervised between giggles. Bumping heads goodbye, his eyes close to mine, he said, "Thank you for letting me make a lovely mess."

I decided that rice would make just as lovely a mess as sand and be easier to clean up. I hated the cleanup work but he so needed the zealous activity that I supplied the rice, and he threw it about just as joyously as he had the sand.

Then, early one morning, David phoned me. There was a phone on the wall of his room; if he wanted to call someone, he would have a nurse dial the number and hold the receiver up to the wall of the bubble. "Friend, we are in trouble. No more lovely messes. A nurse slipped on the rice."

"That can't be, I cleaned up every grain!"

"You did, but when you weren't looking, I hid some in that little car. This morning, I made a mess and she slipped." "Are you all right?"

"Yeah, I got a warning, that's all."

No one mentioned the incident to me.

More mischief: David always loved words, and especially delighted in exploring the forbidden realms of language. He conned me into saying several curse words and the next day said, "Listen. I recorded you."

"David, that was dishonest and could get us in trouble. Everyone is trying to stop your cursing, and what am I doing? I am saying curse words—corrupting you." Without comment, he erased the recording.

"Why do I like to say curse words—do other kids like to say them, too?"
"All kids go through the bathroom stage. They say curse words and giggle."

"What do you mean? Why?"

"Oh, one will say a curse word, and then they all giggle and then the next one will say another curse word, and they giggle again and they keep this up until they get tired of it all, and it's no longer fun. Also, kids learn that saying a curse word upsets grownups; it pushes a button that sends them into orbit—but you discovered that long ago. You've had fun shocking people."

"Could we practice?" he asked. "Sure."

For years we played the curse game—say a bad word, then giggle, giggle. He learned most of his curse words from TV, but some, like "urine head," he made up. I had no explanation for him as to why some words were curse words and, yet, real words—like "damn," "bitch," and "God."

Always, there was the dichotomy. Just as you were becoming convinced that David was progressing normally and had transcended his terribly confining world, something would remind you of how unusual he really was. In the winter, after his fifth birthday, I was sitting on the windowsill and said, "I have to move, my back is getting ice cold."

"What do you mean?"

"It's too cold to sit here. This window is ice cold." "What do you mean, ice cold?"

"Being next to this icy window makes me cold." "You mean, you are ice cold?"

"Yes. I feel cold all over."

"No, no—ice is cold, but you can't feel it." "Of course I can feel cold." "No, no, ice is for Cokes—you can't feel it!"

After more futile arguing I realized that he was not joking, he really did not believe me. His sensory deprivation was mind-boggling—a toddler knew more. I thought: He's five, he's bright. How do I teach cold?

"Okay, kid, I'll prove it to you. You will feel cold." I filled a plastic bag with ice, secured it in two more bags and slipped it under the PVC crib floor. "Sit on it. No, not on your knees, sit on your rear end."

He sat awhile and smirked, "I don't feel anything. I was right! You can't feel cold."

"Just stay put a little longer." All of a sudden, startled, he screeched, "Oh!" He stood up and yelled, "It's still cold!" as he touched his bottom.

David never lost his fascination with ice, and for years we did wonderful things with ice. He watched ice melt, timed how long it took to melt in different sized containers, stuck pencils in a wash basin of ice and watched them "destruct" (fall over). He delighted in throwing ice chips on me. Sometimes when he was in what he termed a "frantic mood," he lay down on bags of ice to relax.

He requested that I bring something else frozen, so I brought a package of frozen green peas. He dumped them from one plastic beaker to another. Sometime later he said, "I sure have waited a long time for those peas to get thin. He did not want to feel a heated, empty pan. "No, no, I learned cold from ice, I have to learn hot from water, too." I warmed some water in the pan, and he stuck his gloved hand in it.

Coming so relatively late in life to an understanding of hot and cold, he tried to make up for lost time, studying them intently—he deduced, "I can tell it's cold and windy outside because people who don't have much clothes on are all hunched over, and the ones that look like they have lots of clothes on walk normal."

We settled hot and cold, but the concept of wind never did completely penetrate. I made a paper windmill to go inside the bubble. He blew on it and put it by a vent to spin, but never generalized this to wind outside. I couldn't adequately explain the wind's rushing force. Then, one night during a violent storm, the lampposts bent and trash blew across the parking lot. He conceded, "You're right, wind is powerful."

Some things like cold, wind, and the feel of fur absolutely cannot be described by words. I found this startling, probably because I had never given it any thought before. But again and again, in my experience with David, I grappled with other jarring, sobering realities of the effects of his deprivation. How many times did I search in vain for words to explain simple things— hills, plumbing, and oil? David thought my fur jacket was beautiful. Touching it through the glove, he looked at me wistfully and questioned, "Would you like for me to be able to really feel that fur?"

"Yes, love."

Unless one had actually spent time in David's quarters it would be virtually impossible to understand his oppressively restricted environment and narrow view of the world. His unique visual/spatial/perceptual development was intriguing but also frustrating, because I could not correct his misconceptions. We spent hours discussing the buildings seen from his window. Nothing I said or did altered his belief that the buildings were flat— just rectangles, parallelograms, and lines.

I drew optical illusions to demonstrate that our perceptions were not necessarily realities. I pointed out, "The bubble portholes are circles. Move to the far corner of the crib and look at one. What is it?"

"Oh my, it's an oval! But it's really a circle."

"Right, David. That's what I'm trying to tell you. We don't always see things as they really are."

Our first model of Fannin Street consisted of silhouettes of each building, painstakingly drawn according to David's instructions and pasted on blue construction paper. "It's perfect and proves that the buildings are flat," he declared.

"If the buildings are just flat, why do people go in them? The hospital front looks flat from the outside, but we are inside. The same with those buildings." He just looked puzzled.

David's unique view of the world led to many requests for Jackie and me to draw what we saw from a window in our house. Attempts to draw a more complex rendering of our homes proved to be incomprehensible to him.

"Don't bother about that," he would say. "Just draw what you can see from one window."

In short, David seemed unable to integrate a more three-dimensional view of the world. His perceptions confirmed what was proclaimed by the eighteenth-century British empiricist, Bishop Berkeley, that judgments made about depth, distance, and space are based entirely on memories of past experiences.

In December, my mother was in adjoining St. Luke's Hospital for two weeks, but not confined to bed. Therefore, she visited with David and me. She reminded him of his great-grandmother; he considered her wise and pretty in her "beautiful robes." He avowed, "Mary, I don't want to hurt your feelings, but if your mother visits me, you can stay at home and work on your house."

I said, "Great, I have so much work with the remodeling." I do not know what they did; I didn't care to know.

David's view: "We had fun."

Mother's view: "He had me hopping—he certainly is bossy." David established rituals for our times together: first, bump heads, then play hide-and-go-seek. Playing hide-and-go-seek was outlandishly ludicrous. Kay Miller started with the silly game of "tent"—a combination of peek-a-boo and hide-and-go-seek. She threw a sheet over the crib and they took turns hiding. Then David decided my hiding was no fun so I became the seeker. After dark, with the lights outs, he hid in the shadows.

If I came early, we ate supper together. If I came at seven, I peeled and ate a grapefruit while he ate pudding. He liked the aroma of grapefruit, which penetrated the air filters. Sometimes, at his request, I fed him pudding. When I left, he was ready to sleep—in pajamas on a fluffy rug with a pillow and Big Bird baby blanket. He drifted to sleep listening to an orchestral recording of Beatles music.

As a little boy, my son, Bill, had been similar to David: he'd had a quick mind, a keen sense of humor, and had been innately artistic. Both, perplexingly moody, were volatile in openly reacting to, or expressing, pleasure or distress. Their ability to become intensely engrossed in an activity made it easy for me to absorb myself in their play and projects.

Things I had done with my son I now did with David—watching clouds, finding beauty in little things. David marveled at pigeons on the ledge "with a thousand colors" and Bill had collected shiny, colored beetles. Although similar in temperament and interests, they were as different as day and night in appearance. Bill, always tall and robust, has blue eyes and red-blond hair. David, slight and slender, had inherited the Mediterranean coloring of his mother, who was of Italian ancestry.

Further, David found change almost intolerable; while my son, who was now a troubleshooter for an engineering firm, thrived on change. When David was five (and Bill was thirty-one), Bill wrote in a letter to me: "'Out' is the best word to describe the way I feel. Distance becomes nothing but an airplane ride—nothing stops me from going where I choose; it is a nice feeling. I relish the changes, the new situations—they fit my personality. I like having to deal with people of totally different cultures and ideas. I find my tolerance for security and stability at a minimum. My security and stability are found in change. Cultural shock is my adrenaline."

David thought my son was great—from faraway places he wrote exciting letters, which could be read and reread. David and I traveled the world with Bill. We sat on a barge in the Persian Gulf. We toured King Ludwig II's Bavarian fairy-tale castle. We retired to Maui to paint.

In many ways, Bill's world was more real and interesting for David than the world beyond Fannin Street or his front yard at home. Bill related comic interactions in script form, and his tale of "The Lost Key in Bahrain," describing two inept workers trying to adjust to Texan ways, captivated David:

"The key for the tool shed was lost. Solution simple—call maintenance and have the lock changed. At eight in the morning, two workers show up.

"'We change lock.' 'Okay, change lock.'

"They take the doorknob off, throw it away. The hole is too little for the new knob. They drill a hole—too big. They cut two boards and nail them over the hole. Stop work, wash their hands, feet, and face, pray, and go back to work. Drill a new hole in the board. Hole is too small, but they spend one hour trying to make the new knob go in anyway. Lunchtime. They come back, drill a larger hole, now the hole is too big. Again, they persist in trying to make the new knob fit. Each time they fail, they stop, wash their hands, feet, face, and pray.

"Back to work. They remove the boards and cut new ones. The foreman, a Texan, completely beside himself at this point, has been watching them from time to time all day, as it is his shed. He grabs the drill, drills the hole the proper size, throws the drill in the ocean and says, 'Now put the #%@*#! doorknob in the hole and give me the keys.' Yes, in the process of the day's work, they had lost the new keys."

David turned Bill's script into a play. Then, using the same theme, he created the first two of a series of plays. In "The Sign Company," the stupid deliveryman never goes to the correct address. In "The Service Station," the attendant puts gas in the "oil tank" and water in the gas tank.

In time, his plays became quite sophisticated. We rehearsed for hours. He directed and gave me acting lessons.

David compulsively ordered his world; he wanted nothing left to chance. Jackie and I both took extreme measures to let him know if we were running late. He once told me, "I never have to wonder about you—Miss Predictable."

The on-again, off-again delivery dates of the space suit accelerated David's apprehension. To his way of thinking, the space suit did not fit into his schedule. A suit, not the whole MBIS unit, finally arrived in September 1976. Having to actually leave the bubble in the MBIS was fast becoming a reality, and he started to worry in earnest.

Even though David was only five, he recognized his difference and dreaded what the future held—limited choices, feelings of alienation, and increased need to be polite and compliant so as not to reveal his anger. He sensed that his growing older was difficult for people and that they were moving away from him. All of this was very frightening, because his very existence was in danger if his caretakers deserted him.

After several weeks of bad dreams, David verbalized two recurring ones: Thousands of spiders attack him; he can kill or ward off the little and the medium-sized spiders, but not the great big spider.

"Make it into a play and change the end," I suggested. He did so; the spiders attacked us and he destroyed the giant spider with a rocket.

But, in an even more disturbing nightmare, the King of Germs dispatched thousands and thousands of wives to invade his bubble. He slew the wives, but the King just married thousands more and sent them after him. No way could he kill the King of Germs. "I wake up screaming and I don't know if it's a bad dream or if they're really pouncing on me," he confided. "Maybe I'm crazy. Maybe I'm losing my mind."

"No, you're not crazy. Let's rewrite this dream." It wasn't easy, but eventually he came up with a play in which he annihilated the King of Germs with a special ray gun. With the King of Germs dead, I appealed to his sense of humor. "Some dreams are silly-crazy," I told him. "I dreamed it was Christmas and everyone wore black and orange Halloween costumes."

He laughed and elaborated on the theme: "It is Christmas, there are miniature Easter baskets and bunnies on the tree. It is Easter and there are tiny Christmas trees in the baskets with the eggs. It is Fourth of July and flags are stuck in pumpkins. It's Easter and we have a pumpkin for a basket." Delighted with himself, he kept the story going for a long time.

David had learned to manage nightmares, but the anguished fear of going crazy plagued him from then on.

6.

THE SPACE SUIT

"It's so quiet in here without the blowers," David said.

"Yes, it's almost eerie. I didn't know you had been talking so loud all these years. Out of the bubble, your voice is different—lower pitched, like a man's almost. When you were five, we thought the constant noise might cause a hearing loss.

"Remember that hearing test—oh, gee! We had so many problems then, the space suit and all."

"Without a doubt, 1977 was an awful year. The immunologist, Dr. Watson, from England was here and told me, 'Someday you must write a book, not about the boy, but all the balmy people around him.'"

"He had a point," said David, laughing.

In January 1977, Donna Curlin was promoted to head nurse, and Brynn Holcomb, R.N., became David's caretaker. Jackie, David, and I now had a new set of problems. Brynn, young, confident, with an appealing smile, had moved to Houston to marry a physician, a trainee under Dr. Nichols. Brynn felt she needed no advice on managing a five-year-old boy. Typically, a young nurse has little authority in a hospital, but Dr. Nichols was so enamored with her that she was allowed many liberties. They needed no one else, not Miss Potts, and certainly not Jackie and me.

David was happy when he returned to the hospital on Saturday after Easter. He made plastic eggs "rain" from an Easter basket "cloud." But, by Thursday, he had marked facial tics and had worked himself into a frenzy over the upcoming hearing test.

"Mary, could I talk to you about something? I'm frightened—I'm going to have a hearing test."

"No need to be frightened; it doesn't hurt."

"No, no, I know about the ear muffs—it's not that. They have to put a wire in. See, they will put it through here and bacteria will come in!"

Saturday night, totally convinced of impending doom, he came back with "Yes, but" to my every comment and beseeched, "You'll be here?"

Without his knowledge, I solicited chief electrician Tom Langford's help. Monday evening, David jovially greeted me with; "Guess what? Mr. Langford is putting the wire in a different way so bacteria can't get inside. Could you please come back tomorrow night? Wednesday morning is the hearing test."

Tuesday night, agitated and. pacing, he said, "I'm worrying—the test and this terrible storm." The claps of thunder and flashes of lightening seemed to be right in the room. "I know you showed me lightning sparks by rubbing your scarf on the bubble, and Mr. Langford promised me that germs couldn't crawl along his wire, but hold me, calm me down, make me feel good." The storm ended and I held him and pressed my hands against his back until he fell asleep.

Comforting David would have been easier if I could have assumed the natural position of placing him on my lap. Holding him with the gloves was backbreaking and physically exhausting. I had to stand squarely erect or half-sit on the edge of a high stool in order to extend my arms into the heavy rubber gloves to embrace him. Very quickly, my arms became numb and. drenched in sweat. David, enfolded in my arms, cuddled comfortably against my chest. Often, he lay flat on his stomach as I pressed my hands against his hips and shoulders. Usually, but not always, after he calmed somewhat, I could sit on the stool with just one hand touching his back.

The test on Wednesday went well; he was calm and had no hearing loss.

But troubles never seemed far away at that time. The next afternoon at five, Nurse Brandy said, "Thank God you are here! David has a stomachache." He described cramps; I convinced him he had gas. After awhile the pain subsided and we played. Early the next morning he said, "Mary, we sure had us a problem last night—didn't we?"

The next week went no better. The observing psychoanalyst brought a photographer. His visits upset David, but this time he screamed, "I hate him, he has mean eyes!"

The climax of this difficult time came on Friday, May 19, 1977. NASA hooked the MBIS flange on the supply bubble; David would exit through this into the suit. When I walked in, he was lying down, kicking and sobbing. The nurse flung up her arms, declaring, "I've tried everything!" and gladly left, closing the door.

"All right, David, sit up and let's talk," I said quietly. Snuggling close in my arms he whimpered, "Lillie doesn't understand what an awful day I had.

First the space suit came. Indiana is ruined and Texas is curled up!" (Urine had overflowed the potty onto his U.S.A. map.) Finally, he settled down and even laughed, but the facial tics never diminished.

The space suit created lots of excitement and exuberance. I remained somewhat positive because of the three impressive men from NASA: Bill Carmean, Paul Ferguson, and Dick Graves. They interacted with David in a sensitive manner and seemed dedicated to expanding his world. Although David dreaded entering the suit, he enjoyed talking with these men. They gave him fabulous space pictures which years later he still treasured.

The space suit called for many meetings to decide logistics, security, legal issues, and how to deal with the news media. The attorneys wanted to know who would be responsible in the event of an accident.

One of the biggest questions was, "Where does he go?" In vain, I pushed for David's wish, quoting what he had told me: "I would like to go in the parking lot to look at my window, and open car doors and the gate."

But the parking lot was vetoed—crowds would descend, he might get hurt or damage the suit. No one except Dr. Desmond listened to my reasoning: that David was only five and very frightened, and needed an incentive to cooperate—such as his choice of space suit destinations.

I was already abject and worn to a frazzle when the final blow fell. Dr. Nichols announced the first space suit donning was to be a gala event with VIPs and the major networks invited. I could not imagine anything more frightening for David, but was overruled. I even expressed concern to Carol Ann and David Sr., but they anticipated no problems.

On May 27, the day David went home, my son called from the airport, "Your favorite escort is here. Is the retirement party for Dr. Blattner (chairman of Pediatrics and physician-in-chief at TCH) still on?" Bill told Dr. Larry Tabor, "Mother is stressed out, what she needs is a night out on the town."

I was so stressed at this point that I actually got drunk for the first time in my life, as I poured out my frustrations to my son at Cody's, a Houston nightspot.

"Nurses order me around, people ignore my concerns; I'm stomped on and humiliated. Everyone is bitching, 'You're over-involved.' In my profession, personal and emotional involvement is taboo, but then no one ever taught me how to help a boy survive in a bubble."

"Mother, you're wasting time and energy being miserable. Stop it. Forget other people, make decisions, charge ahead. Help David to trust, let him learn by discovery and figure out a better environment. Maybe you can house him at NASA. I can see him going off into space, doing something tremendous. He's perfect for it, he could tolerate the isolation. Teach him math, astronomy, and physics, and all mankind will profit."

At my home, Bill opened the door: One step inside and the living room floor came up to hit me. For two days, I nursed my first and last hangover; David's problems were held in abeyance.

In years to come, Bill held onto fantasies of my ability to fashion a pleasant and satisfying world for David. To him it seemed so easy.

Once my confidence returned, my priority was to squelch the headline making festivities. Trying to make Dr. Nichols understand David's fears was a waste of time, so I casually remarked, "It might be embarrassing, with the network cameras going, when he has a tantrum and refuses to get in the suit." The next thing I knew, the entire VIP spectacle had been canceled and only the TCH camera crew, headed by James de Leon, would be present.

David returned on July 12, after a trip home, and talked of nothing except antagonism about the space suit. I put forth every conceivable incentive, but he remained adamantly opposed.

"I don't want to go to another room! I don't want to look out of another window to see the parking lot exit!"

"You have mixed feelings. It's exciting and it's scary, too, but so is anything new or strange."

"No, I'm not frightened, I'm just down about it all. Will you be here? Please, I want you here."

"I'll be here, your parents will be here, and they have been trained to operate it." Finally, I hit on something that piqued his interest. "You can see the ice machine, push the handle, and get ice!"

But he was far from completely persuaded. "I've decided there are two kinds of people—ones you can trust and ones you can't trust, and I only know two people I trust—you and Mr. Langford," he said.

I agreed that some people can't be trusted, but added, "You can trust the NASA men; Dick Graves is a Ph.D. microbiologist, and both engineers work on spaceships. Your suit has two backup systems—it's safe, those three men can handle any problem, and your father knows how it works."

We talked to David's parents on the phone, but their zeal for Friday didn't rub off on him. His mother told me, "You're the only person my son invited."

David's last word on the subject was, "I'm not going in the space suit. I'm just going to try it out, and then they are going to disconnect it and take it away."

The space suit had a unique origin. It exemplifies the idea that David's situation was utterly new and required the kind of creative thinking at which kids excel, but that often eludes educated adults. It was a suggestion included in a letter from a twelve-year-old boy who had apparently read one of the early media reports regarding the Bubble Boy. Sue Criswell, a Baylor fellow in microbiology working in the NASA lab, presented the idea to Fred Spross, the project engineer for NASA's Biological Isolation Garments (BIGs). He and the other bright engineers were enthusiastic.

The space suit that began as a "fun project" in the garages of NASA engineers was now a reality, after enormous effort. Paul Ferguson, a NASA flight engineer, told me, "We didn't imagine all the problems—cost, engineering, and legal. There was no room for error. Nothing was simple—we worked our tails off, mostly on our own time."

Bill Carmean, of Martin Marietta, prepared the requirements and Paul Ferguson was charged with quality control and working out the mechanical and electrical systems. Within a year, the MBIS was built. Then followed a year of hassles over responsibility—was it test hardware or medical equipment? Because nurses were involved, it was designated medical equipment. Then they started all over because David had grown taller.

Although David's suit resembled the astronauts' pressurized life support systems, the prototype was the Apollo BIGs worn by the returning lunar astronauts before they went into quarantine to protect earth from possible harmful moon pathogens.

But David's suit was even more problematic. As Dr. Graves pointed out, "David's coming from a sterile environment and going into a sterile environment was more complex than the BIGs. Once the MBIS with a child inside is taken into the unsterile outside world, how do you get him out of the suit and back into sterile living quarters without contaminating him or the inside of the suit? You can't bring him and the suit back into the bubble."

It was determined that David would enter and exit the suit by the same process as supplies went in and trash came out of the bubble. A ten-foot-long by eighteen-inch-diameter yellow tunnel was attached to the back of the suit. The other end had a metal-disc door, which connected to a port on the supply. One problem was that the porthole was so high from the floor that David would have to stand on a chair to exit or enter the tunnel. Precarious indeed.

Once he was in the suit, the tunnel would be collapsed by zipping a sheath over it and forcing the sterile air back into the bubble. Then the port hole inside the supply would be sealed off, the disk closed, disconnected, and mounted on the cart that would follow David around—it consisted of a power unit and blower mounted on a lawnmower chassis. Positive air pressure kept the suit ballooned so that, if punctured, outside air could not enter. Air blew into the helmet, and out of vents at the ankles.

The NASA men had been training the parents and two nurses to operate the mobile unit since before Christmas. From my viewing of the NASA film one year ago, the small gloves were the most promising feature. At five years and ten months of age, David, for the first time, easily would be able to pick up something not sterilized.

The day before the scheduled event, David had a terrifying experience: A CRC patient unlatched, but did not open, the playroom door. His anxiety escalated, as he feared that, perhaps, germs had come in through the unlatched door.

At eleven o'clock, Friday, July 29, 1977, three NASA men, David's parents, Katherine, Jackie, Nichols, two nurses, the MBIS, a camera crew, and public relations personnel packed into his quarters. If one person wanted to move, a half dozen others had to move first. Jackie and I were between the window and the crib with David. His father, the crowd, and the MBIS were on the other side of the room between the playroom and hall door.

David demanded, "Mary, in the gloves—please hold me!" It was a three-ring circus. When the countdown started, he huddled in my arms as far away from the MBIS as possible.

"I don't believe all this. Mary, can you believe all this? Look at that thing on the end of the tunnel. Now that is what I'm afraid of. Germs could come in there."

"No, David, they won't. Those men know their job, they have practiced. Trust them."

"What is that book they're reading?"

"It's the operating manual—a checklist to avoid errors. One reads, two do. Nothing is left to chance."

"Would you ask them to let me see it?"

"I'll read—'Optimizing Procedures and Maintenance'." "Turn to the last page. Oh my God, fifty-four pages of written instructions! Are they gonna read all that?"

"YES."

"It's a nice day and everything is going right—isn't it? Mary, will you be here at seven tonight?"

"For the hundredth time, yes."

"Son, it's time to go in," said his father.

"Come on, remember, you'll visit the ice machine and Potsy's kitchen. Everything will be fine, you will have fun," I said.'

"Okay, I'll go when the clock says twenty (12:20). It's twenty, I'll go when it says twenty-five—I'll wait till thirty—I'll go at forty."

David was pathetic, trembling. As I tried to alleviate his terror, Dr. Nichols, standing next to me, took my hand.

"You're so nervous, you're shaking," he whispered. "He'll never move with all these people watching," I whispered back. I wanted to say, "I told you so, and you'd shake too if you had been standing and holding him for an hour and a half." He cleared the room, but many faces stared from the hall. We had total silence.

David asked me, "Is it okay?"

"Yes."

He crawled into the tunnel, head first, but quickly returned.

"Look," I said, "If you crawl head first you've got to do a flip to put your feet in first: Then sit up and bend forward to get your head in the helmet." Down the tunnel again, he turned and correctly flipped into the right position, but his head stuck. He let out a bloodcurdling scream and scampered back. I felt a surge of nausea. I explained what he was doing wrong, and he tried again. On the fifth attempt he called back, "Mary, it would be better if you were down here."

I didn't move until everyone shouted, "Get down there!" In one second he flipped, and I popped his head down and into the helmet. After he had his hands in the gloves, he stuck them up in front of his face and grinned from ear to ear.

"I like it!" he said, beaming.

The cameras were filming my back, not David with his mother; the photographers angrily bellowed at me to get out of the way. I smelled something burning, looked up, and saw that the floodlights mounted near the playroom had caught it on fire. (It was quickly extinguished.) I was utterly depleted, a rumpled mess with two sopping wet sleeves.

Standing on the chair and supported by his parents, David tired during the tedious thirty-minute wait to be disconnected from the isolator. Lowered to the floor, he lost his balance and could hardly walk. Yet he staggered across the hall and down about four steps from his door to the ice machine. He filled a cup with ice. He saw his favorite nurse, Dorothy, at the end of the hall and propelled himself forward to hand her the ice. His face radiated joy. For the first time, he had handed an object to another person.

That evening David excitedly said, "Working the ice machine and carrying a cup of ice to Dorothy was the most fun." Fatigued, he was willing to go to bed early. Never before had he taken more than six steps in one direction; today, he had walked at least thirty feet. So far he had voiced no objections to a second excursion scheduled for the next Friday.

On Monday evening, I heard him crying before I entered his room. "I'll get ice, and you lie on it awhile, and then tell me all about it," I said.

"It's been a horrible, horrible day and it's all NASA's fault—the flange for the suit had to stay on, and the acid puddled in the sleeve and won't dissipate."

"Stay put on the ice until I get the acid mopped up so you can uncap the crib and get your food. It's been a bad luck day. Let's just start all over."

He settled down and decided to eat, but the food box was locked and the nurses lost the piece of paper with the combination. I found it in a wastebasket. "David, memorize it," I insisted. "Now, no more tantrums over the lock."

All was quiet when the nurse returned, and David announced, "We have everything under control."

"You should love Mary a lot," she said. "What would you do without her?"

He frowned. "We never discuss loving each other," I said quietly.

A few days later, he said, "You are the only person I know who doesn't say I love you. You do love me? I know you love me. You do love me—don't you?"

Somewhat taken aback, I spoke carefully. "Well, I believe actions count—words are easy to say, and so many people pop in and say I love you. I know some of them really do love you, but for others, it's like saying hello or goodbye."

Several weeks later, trying to comfort him, I said, "Love, listen...."

He interrupted, "Do you know what you called me? 'Love.' You said I was 'love.' "

Over the years, on very special occasions, I did call him "love."

The next day, Carol Ann attended the CDP meeting. She then viewed the films of David in his space suit, while I ate lunch with him. When she joined us, she expressed disappointment, saying that David looked "rather sad" in many of the pictures.

Later, David discussed his reservations about getting in the suit again. I told him, "You'll have fun." I explained that Susan Thurber, the physical therapist, would teach him to walk better so that he could play down in CDP.

When I went to speak with Dr. Nichols about David's anxiety, he stopped me before I finished the first sentence. "I don't have time for housekeeping details. The problem is you're an old hen with one chick."

"You're so right," I sharply retorted. "And something tells me this particular chick needs an old hen." A hole in the suit cancelled the Friday excursion.

Dr. Ralph D. Feigin, the new chairman of the Department of Pediatrics of Baylor and physician-in-chief at TCH arrived in the middle of July 1977, and immediately made his presence known to everyone from section heads to parking lot attendants. Jackie described him as "a man with an incredibly organized mind who is impatient with nonessentials or people who cannot quickly express or articulate. He has no time for people who can't put their ideas into focus and work toward a goal." This young man, not yet forty, impressed me as being dynamic, brilliant, and decisive. I felt he conveyed authority and trust.

The first week in August, Dr. Desmond called me to her office to discuss David's emotional state with Dr. Feigin. I was succinct: "He's overanxious, I'm not sure he can continue. I believe it's a question of time. We are looking at either psychological or physical death."

He appeared stunned. "Everyone keeps saying he is doing so well."

I explained to Dr. Feigin that this was an example of the ongoing misperception of David as the Happy Bubble Boy. It seemed to me that this illusion had two causes. First, David presented a happy face to most people because he knew he depended on others utterly for his survival, and he feared alienating them. Second, the idea that he was doing poorly in his confinement was simply too much for people to bear, so they chose to believe he was happy.

I, however, was in a unique position. He trusted me enough to show me his unhappy side, and I have always been a hardheaded realist, unable to fool myself into believing a situation is positive when it is not.

Dr. Feigin looked directly at me; he could see that I was serious. "I promise I will do something." He paced for a few minutes and walked back to me. "I'll contact all the eminent immunologists."

Weeks later he came to me. "I am sorry—I talked at length with leading immunologists. They have nothing to offer." David's confinement would have to continue indefinitely. I was devastated, but not surprised. I had stayed with the here-and-now in relating to David, so I had never got caught up in the hope of a cure tomorrow.

The extensive publicity surrounding the space suit created problems. Government funds were getting tight, and it was difficult to justify so much of the taxpayers' money being spent on one child. Criticisms of dehumanization by technology came from both the medical community and the public. Loony, and often frightening, letters with miraculous cures, accusations, or threats to "free the prisoner" flooded the hospital.

We carried on. Friday evening, August 12, David had a cricket in a tiny bamboo box—the cricket was caught in the hospital; I don't know who gave him the box. He announced, "I've been waiting for you before I kill it. Put it in a bag of ice, and I'll stomp on it." With some misgivings, I complied. He jumped and jumped, but missed each time. It appeared dead, but back in its box it came to life.

"Crickets are good luck," I said, "Let me put it in a bush outside." "No, put it in a cup of ice and cover it with plastic so it won't pop out.

Get another cricket. The hospital is full of them. Go look."

Sunday evening, when my mother went with me to see David, he was in a choleric mood. "The problem is the space suit," she theorized. "The thought of a little freedom is upsetting him—he's afraid if he learns what he's missing, life will be intolerable."

Carol Ann had expressed similar fears, "What if he refuses to go back in the bubble?"

On this visit, my mother encountered David's grotesquely minuscule friend, J.J., a twelve-month-old CRC patient. Walking to the elevator she said, "I nearly fainted when I saw that poor child."

J.J. was a failure to thrive child who weighed only five pounds. I had warned my mother about his unique appearance. "You did," she said, "but still I wasn't prepared to see an infant with an old man's face; that smile with a mouthful of teeth. David seems fond of him."

"Yes, J.J. spends a lot of time with us. We move the wastebasket out and put his swing there—he watches and smiles."

During David's next hospital stay, a lot of commotion centered around the so-called "devil baby." Tales had spread that the hospital was harboring a red-skinned baby with horns who supposedly cursed the doctors at birth. Local TV stations and the *Houston Chronicle* on October 6, 1977, reported the rumors. People, mostly from Louisiana, flocked to the hospital. Many support people refused to work on the third floor where he was supposedly kept. One night as I left late, a group approached me, "Did you see him? Wasn't that you by the third floor window?"

Apparently, people believed David's tiny, frail friend, J.J. was the notorious "devil baby". Two armed guards were assigned to CRC to protect David from someone searching for the devil. David enjoyed conversing with the guards and took it upon himself to set visitors straight: " J.J. is just J.J. He doesn't curse. He can't talk." After several weeks, the fury over the "devil baby" ended. J.J., oblivious to it all, continued to spend time with us.

On October 13, the night before David was to get in the space suit for the second time, he rocked, sucked his thumb, twitched, and finally admitted, "I'm afraid about tomorrow—the germs—and I don't know why else I'm afraid."

I tried to be reassuring. "This time is going to be fun. We'll go down to CDP. I promise, if you do exactly what is asked for the first minutes while they film you with the teacher, you can play ball with Katherine, write on the blackboard, and use a pencil."

After some mulling over, he said, "Okay, but could I ask you a favor? Please come at seven tomorrow night. It's not your night, but please be here."

The next morning Dr. Desmond went with me to see him. He was still in his pajamas and trying to eat breakfast. When I said I would come back later, he became agitated and desperately pleaded, "Hold me, hold me!"

But that particular space suit experience went well. I encouraged him to throw a ball to his sister; when she threw it back, he had an infant-like startle. It occurred to me that he had never seen an object flying through the air in his direction before.

Thursday, the night before the third space suit excursion, David was somewhat apprehensive, but when the hour came, he had a good time: he threw beanbags, slammed doors, and hugged his mother. His balance was now good, and he walked the entire distance back to the elevator.

Carol Ann confided, "You give my son courage. You gave him the courage to get into the space suit the first time. Thank you."

That evening, David was calm, like a different child—jovial and playful. He was in a give-and-take mood and immediately announced, "Tonight I'm going to manipulate you." We played with the big blocks from CDP and went through our rituals. It had been a happy, happy day. He asked, "Why do you let me manipulate you?"

"Because I like to see the wheels turning in your head and see how clever you are."

At half past seven, I was ready to leave, and he suddenly started making demands—get a puzzle, find a certain record, on and on. Exasperated, I said, "No more!" He threw himself down, crying. "Come on, David, you are ruining what has been a perfect evening. I have to go."

"Look at the clock!" he said, laughing loudly. "I kept you ten minutes longer. How is that for manipulation?"

Just then his mother called. David told her, "I had fun today, and I'm having fun right now. I'm happy."

She then spoke to me, very distraught. She'd lost a gift, a special rosary, from the bishop. She didn't want David to know.

Very early Saturday morning, I went back to pick up a book purposely left so I could look for the rosary in daylight. "You're not going to find that rosary around here—she had it in her hand when she walked out." So much for secrets. I retraced her steps and went to lost-and-found as well as the chaplain's office. Somehow finding the rosary was the most important thing in the world. Our unspoken fear—its loss was an ominous sign.

I called Carol Ann. She had hoped I would find the rosary. She then expressed distress at David's picture being in the paper with an article by the observing psychoanalyst. "He is exploiting my son. I've been afraid to say anything, but I wanted you to know how I feel."

"Carol Ann, you have the right to express opinions. You always say you defer to the professionals because they know what is best. But you are his mother; act on your judgments and have faith in your instincts. You're right about this, four articles in four weeks is too much. You son has vehemently expressed his dislike of the man. I object because the taping, picture taking, and questioning agitate David." The pain over the loss of the rosary and this frank discussion marked the beginning of a warm, close relationship between Carol Ann and me.

Dr. Nichols rightly demanded that the professionals involved with David adhere to hospital and Baylor protocols. The psychoanalyst opted to contact Carol Ann directly, rather than go through the stringent TCH and Baylor human research protocols. She did not respond to his request for a note indicating that she was aware of his efforts and approved of their continuation. The psychoanalyst's observations ceased.

Searching for the rosary, I met an Episcopalian priest who had tried, at Carol Ann's request, to give David religious instruction. He wanted to try again and asked if I would convince David to let him in the room. After encouragement from Carol Ann, I broached the subject with David. He said, "No!" but later that evening, "I changed my mind. If you come and stay for the first lesson, I'll do it."

Everything was set for late in the afternoon. The priest came equipped with interesting puppets; David was charming and receptive. But the priest, standing between the window and the crib, turned white and froze, unable to do anything. I had witnessed similar reactions from other people entering David's quarters—the realization that David was confined to such a tiny space was simply too much for many people to bear.

After he left, David laughed. "I kept my promise, so now I have you for an extra hour."

Religious training for David was important to both his mother and me. To her chagrin, the priest and nun in Conroe had not established rapport with David. "You and I will teach him," she finally proclaimed.

"I'm not Roman Catholic."

"The difference between Episcopalian and Catholic doesn't matter. I trust you to teach my son the right thing."

I didn't accomplish much reading to him, but he listened to my telling Old Testament stories. I concluded that a child needs the ambiance of a church and the camaraderie of catechism classes to appreciate the rituals of the church.

David had facial tics, and his thumb sucking now included vigorous rubbing of the bridge of his nose with his index finger. At times, the skin between his eyes was scraped raw. He complained of being nervous, but didn't or couldn't verbalize why.

Brynn, alarmed by his behavior and generalized twitching, decided the TV program, *Emergency*, was the source of his anxiety. I disagreed, even though I didn't approve of many of the programs he watched. I thought the complexities of his life were defeating him.

Tuesday night he pleaded, "Hold me, calm me. I don't know why I'm so nervous. Please come back tomorrow night. Thursday is your night to be here, come then too. Please, I go home Friday. Always come the night before I go home."

Thursday night, when I walked in, he cried, "There's a big crack in the crib, check for escaping air!" Nurse Brandy and I struggled with it—the crack was merely a crease. "Hold me... I'm frantic... I'm going crazy!" David moaned. The next morning, I was glad to see him off. He had a skeleton costume for Halloween, his favorite holiday.

David's being home didn't help me as much as I had hoped. I had a terrible time with myself in November. I was so enmeshed with him that I couldn't separate my anxieties from his. I had two repeated nightmares:

We are all in a garden and David's space suit goes up in flames. He doesn't seem to be hurt. The parents and those involved with him stand in shock. I grab him and run to the street to hail a taxi. He sits on my lap crying and I reassure him we are on our way to the hospital. I remember I have cold sores—with horror I realize my virus will be fatal to him.

Then David, in the suit, and I are on a platform in the middle of a beautiful lake, like one I knew as a child in Missouri. People on the shore are watching. He and I hold hands and jump in. We swim around, laugh, and have fun. For some reason, I always stay between him and the people on the shore. Then we're back on the platform, but this time it is very high, and we're afraid to jump, but we must. We hold hands and jump into the water, but strangers are pulling at the suit and ripping it, and we're surrounded by attacking fish. I push the people and fish away. Although I'm a good swimmer, I have trouble keeping him afloat. I look to the shore; no one offers to come in the water to help us.

Dr. Desmond had lost much of her objectivity after seeing David so frantic with fear. "Last Friday, I saw how David got strength and security from you, but he is draining you. You cannot be so involved. You will crack up." I appreciated the concern but resented her and the assistant CDP director believing I was so fragile. I replied, "I can't pull out and live with myself."

I attended a press conference on November 3, 1977, Dr. Desmond recounted several of my anecdotes, Drs. Feigin and Nichols emphasized the educational value of the space suit.

As the NASA men demonstrated the MBIS, some reporters looked perplexed or teary; no doubt their illusions of the space suit giving David freedom were shattered. No one asked a question that would dispel the myth of The Happy Bubble Boy. The only cutting questions concerned money.

As David approached school age, there was considerable controversy over how he would be taught. Dr. Nichols and Brynn wanted a teacher to be with David all day. Arden Richardson refused, "No child has a teacher one-to-one all day, and working with him is exhausting." Arden had funds to build a small sterile room at the school for David, and she invited us to tour the special education campus.

On November 17, 1977, Jackie, Brynn, and I met Carol Ann at Arden's office. She made it clear that David's education was the business of the parents and professionals, not a young, know-it-all nurse. Initially, I thought the whole idea of David's attending school was too far out. But Arden's plan seemed plausible. His curriculum would include adaptive physical education and time with a psychologist.

After the meeting, several severely retarded and handicapped children recognized me and came running to hug me. Afterward, Carol Ann said, "I couldn't bear to look at those pitiful children. You held them and talked with them as if nothing were wrong. I have to admire you."

"I'm accustomed to it; it's my job," I said. "I'm not sure I could handle dying children as Jackie does."

David returned on November 29. The hospital had a six-hour power shortage and his little friend, J.J., died early that morning. When I walked in, David said, "J.J. is dead." Before I had a chance to say anything, David asked, "Why didn't you sigh and say ooh, ooh, when I told you J.J. was dead?"

"I don't know."

"Well, that's what everybody says when you tell them somebody's dead. He is dead. It's not good to be dead. I don't want to believe he's dead. And what's more, I'm not buying that stuff about him being up there flying with angels. He is just dead. Dead. Dead. Did you ever know a boy who died? Did you call an ambulance? Did you cry? Oh, it's awful to be dead! Did they call an ambulance when God died?"

"You mean when Jesus died? No, there were none then." "Not even one ambulance?" He sobbed. "It's awful!"

"Stop crying and listen. When I was your age, I felt the same way, but now that so many people I loved have died, death doesn't seem fearful. There is life and there is death, it is all the same process, a cycle. We don't understand the meaning of life so we can't understand death. But life is beautiful, and therefore, I believe death too must be beautiful in a way that we really don't understand. Death is mysterious."

"It can't be good that J.J. is dead."

"You are sad, and I am sad; we will miss him so much, but maybe death for J.J. is not bad. He's been sick and in pain for a long time; death ends pain.

That has to be good. The body dies, but the person we love will always be alive in our hearts and our memories."

"Then love never dies."

"That's right, love is always now. J.J. will have beautiful memories too—his last one will be of Jackie singing as she rocked him."

The attorney vetoed Dr. Desmond's plan for the fourth MBIS excursion to a nearby private garden. Brynn and Dr. Nichols decided David should go to the carpenter shop. Jackie, Dr. Desmond, and I adamantly objected. If the parking lot was too dangerous, what about the sharp scraps on the shop floor? They dismissed our arguments—David needed to understand and respect tools and to identify with his father's interests.

The night before the excursion was one of excruciating agony for David and for me. The minute I walked in he wailed, "Calm me, I'm in a frantic mood." He made half-hearted attempts to play, but quickly reverted to rocking and thumb sucking. He expressed the usual concerns—the tunnel might tear, and so forth.

"I'm not afraid of the carpenter's shop. I don't know why I'm afraid or what I'm afraid of. I must be crazy. Please, please stay until I'm asleep."

He didn't go to sleep until after two o'clock. He lay on his sheepskin bed. I pressed both hands against his back. For hours, with numb, wet arms, I alternated between sitting on the stool and standing. When I realized my blouse was wet from tears, I sobbed aloud, musing, "Am I crying for him or am I crying for me? It hurts so much."

The next morning, in CDP, David walked to me, "Gee, that was some night we had, wasn't it?"

Later in the day I checked on him, and he grinned and said, "I'm okay and they didn't even cut off my head with a saw." I berated myself: Why hadn't I put two and two together last night? His egocentricity—why go to the carpenter's shop if no one planned to do something to or with him? At that moment, I gave serious thought to killing both Nichols and Brynn.

Music lessons, I reasoned, would help to keep David occupied. Drake Mabry, a graduate student in music at Rice University, impressed me as being the perfect teacher. Drake questioned me at length about David's preferences and was pleased to learn his favorite record was the orchestral arrangement of Beatles tunes. Drake selected and purchased a recorder—simple to play and it could go into the bubble.

Drake quickly won David over. He never got very far with the recorder lessons, but they became great friends. He taught David an appreciation for music.

I love music, but have no musical talent. I met with Drake several times; he taught me how to listen, and I too gained a new appreciation of music.

One night when I walked in, David said, "Don't talk. I'm writing music." It was enchanting to watch him "write music" with a marker and a large piece of paper as he listened to music.

The evenings in December were truly happy times. We listened to the Beatles and watched the beautiful sunsets. The pigeons gathered at the windows to eat the bread Potsy had furnished. After dark, he would lie down in the crib and I on the windowsill so we could gaze at the stars as we listened to music.

One evening, David said, "Let's pretend. Let's pretend we're holding hands and walking up the sidewalk to your house. Would you like to do that?"

"Yes, David, I would like to do that. I can't think of anything I would want to do more."

"Oh, Mary, me too. That would really be nice, to be holding hands and walking up to your house. Don't you wish we really could?"

"Yes, love, I do."

7.

DAVID ENTERS GRADE ONE

"Mary, I'm so tired, there is not one part of my body that doesn't hurt. I wish we were back home on Fannin Street. You know what we'd be doing— exercising or playing hide-and-go-seek."

In January 1978, NASA sterilized two new items—a mechanical pencil and an exercise mat. Susan Thurber wanted the mat to facilitate exercise. David seldom used it for that, but he loved to roll up in it and hide. Probably nothing pleased David more than the pencil, and within a few months, Dr. Dick Graves found a way to sterilize an eraser.

An admirer sent David a twenty-five-dollar check, and I requested he be given the money to do with as he pleased. I showed him the check and said, "I'll get it cashed at the bank. Do you want ones or fives?"

"What do you mean ones or fives?"

"I mean one-dollar bills or five-dollar bills."

"No, no, I don't want bills, I want real money—coins. Go now so I can watch you cross Fannin Street."

When I returned, he asked, "Where is the money?" In my purse."

"It can't be. It has to be in a bag like when they rob a bank." At age six, he had never actually seen money, much less had any.

Despite my assurances that bills and coins were equal, David retained his love for the latter. But two valuable coins that had been sterilized and put in the bubble caused problems for weeks.

On March 30, 1978, in a *Houston Post* article titled "Bubble Boy Gulps Coins, Passes Crisis," Dr. Feigin explained the incident. Pragmatic Frank Weaver, BCM public relations, demanded the story be released before the press discovered it and concluded that we were hiding something.

At home on Thursday, January 19, 1978, he swallowed two of these coins, and one lodged in his throat. The most solid food he had was meat sticks, and they were not dense enough to dislodge the coin. The pain became unbearable. He had to return to the hospital on Saturday so a gastroenterologist could push the coin on down with a flexible endoscope. David was given tranquilizers but no general anesthetic for fear of a reaction they could not handle without taking him out of the bubble.

"It was the worst experience of my career," Dr. William Klish told me. "It was terrible to do the procedure with just a light application of four percent tyclocaine spray. We did it in Cooley's amphitheater and when we started lots of people were watching. After David's screams, they scattered—the room was empty. We had no choice but to continue. The problem was he couldn't stay still."

It all happened without my knowledge. I learned of the incident from a colleague on Monday morning; her source of information had been a hospital administrator at a cocktail party.

I rushed upstairs and asked, "David, why didn't you have someone call me?"

"So much was going on, and I slept most of Sunday."

That evening he explained. "It was awful. Boy, was I stupid. Katherine had popcorn—she threw it up in the air and then caught it in her mouth—I tried it with coins. Let me tell you something. Never, never, again will I hold my mouth open and look up at the same time!" Carol Ann spent a lot of time with David the next week. She told me, "I wanted to call you, but didn't want to bother you and ruin your weekend."

Dr. Feigin himself kept close watch on David during this period. A scratch or wound from the coins posed a grave danger. The bacteria that remained harmless in David's digestive tract would be potentially fatal if it invaded his bloodstream. He had a slight fever and tests showed non-virulent bacteria in his blood. He was given oral synthetic penicillin as a precaution. The bacteria that remained harmless in David's digestive tract would be potentially fatal if introduced to the bloodstream. He had a slight fever and tests showed non-virulent bacteria in his blood. He was given oral synthetic penicillin as a precaution. He was fine except for a miserable time with diarrhea. On February 3, he passed the two coins, a 1907 U.S. nickel and an Australian one-cent piece.

Dr. Nichols had phoned Dr. South for advice. I was livid at him for not having called Jackie or me as we could have helped David through the ordeal. On Monday, Dr. Nichols called Dr. Desmond to complain about David's behavior and panic during the procedure. He described David's "marked anxiety characterized by thumb sucking, scraping his forehead, and rocking."

He told the parents David needed psychiatric help. This, too, infuriated me. I wouldn't argue against his needing help, but I didn't think it fair to base this decision on David's reaction to what would have been a traumatic procedure for any six-year-old child.

Dr. Douglas Hansen, a child psychiatrist, began attending the CDP meetings. Dr. Desmond was "greatly relieved to have a psychiatrist on board." Dr. Hansen's explanations of Freud and Piaget's stages of development were informative to Dr. Desmond and the nurses. He was of absolutely no help to Jackie and me. In time, we resented his arrogant attitude toward us and felt he viewed us as over involved, doting alarmists.

David, anxious about the space suit excursion that was scheduled for Friday, February 10, 1978, didn't want to be left alone. On Wednesday evening he phoned. "I'm bored. Could you come over? You promised—if I needed you. Do you have much homework?" When I arrived, he was pacing and tense.

"Mother is coming at six o'clock tomorrow night to ease my pre-flight anxiety, but I don't want to be alone now, and the nurses are busy. They have very completely sick patients on the floor. Will you be here at seven Friday evening and maybe come see me a little bit tomorrow?"

"Yes and yes."

Friday morning Mildred came to my office with a guard. "Trouble, come quick!"

David, in the space suit, was backed into the corner of the elevator gripping the handrail and yelling, refusing to get off. "I want to ride up and down and watch the doors open!" he shouted. It was a hilarious scene: this six-year-old kid, surrounded by Ph.D.s and M.D.s, holding them all at bay. They dared not touch him, let alone yank him off, for fear of damaging the suit.

Dr. Feigin, watching the fiasco, approached me, "Mary, do something about that behavior."

I worked at keeping a straight face, and for the first and only time I threatened David: "Okay, kid, life is a two-way street. Get off this elevator, or I don't visit at seven tonight." He looked at me, grinned, stood straight, and trotted off.

When we passed the "window" (the hospital's double doors), he pleaded to go outside, but that was not part of the arrangement for this excursion. In CDP he opened cabinet doors, flushed the toilet, turned on the faucets in the washbowl, and asked, "Why two faucets?" He was particularly intrigued with the drinking fountain and making the water squirt.

Dr. Nichols was out of town, so Dr. Desmond was in charge of the trip, and she agreed to let him go to the underground garage to look at cars. My schedule did not allow me to accompany him.

That evening he inquired, "Mary, what's this business about a two-way street?"

"Look at Fannin Street," I said. "All the cars going south are on one side and the ones going north are on the other side. Everyone lives by rules. Living is like a two-way street."

"Well, I don't see why cars can't go on either side, either way."

"Think about it. What would happen if the cars drove both ways on both sides? They'd crash. Everybody has to live by rules. It's courtesy, and it's necessary. We have to trust that people will live by rules."

"I thought I was the only person in the whole world that had rules." "No one has complete freedom to do as they please. People have to trust what others will do. I'd be afraid to drive or even go outside the building if I didn't believe that others would do as they're supposed to. Still, I understand how difficult it is for you to be confined and have so many people telling you what you must do. You probably have more rules than most kids."

"You do understand. I'm not allowed to say what I want to do. Like I get in the mobile isolator, and I'm all ready to go, and then I really can't go anyplace—I wanted to go out that window and I couldn't. Tell me again why there are two faucets on the washbowl. I don't see why you need one for hot and one for cold. Water is water!"

The next evening, a Saturday, my mother sent him an African violet with many buds. I explained that the buds would soon become blossoms; probably one would blossom tomorrow. The next day he phoned, "The violet shell didn't crack like you said it would."

"Give it time." Miraculously, the violet bloomed and bloomed, it thrived sitting on the air conditioner in the hot sun.

On February 21, Brynn requested a meeting with Susan, Jackie, and me to discuss David's "bad, sassy, and irritating behavior." Sue and Jackie, both more vocal and patient than me, tried to explain normal six-year-old behavior. They stressed the need for Brynn to let Carol Ann exert more control and take on a mother role rather than her present visitor role. Jackie urged Brynn to read *Children the Challenge*.

The attorneys and the public relations people, as well as the usual group, were involved in more strategy meetings on the upcoming space-suit trip to David's home on February 24, his first outdoor excursion. Weather might be a problem. The temperature had to be between seventy and eighty degrees and there could be no rain. The plan was to allow David to explore the bedroom, bathroom, kitchen, and laundry of his home in Conroe and, weather permitting, to walk completely around the outside of the house in order to experience four dimensions. The group regarded the latter activity, which I had requested, as ridiculous—of course David knew a house had four sides.

I had told David he could play with the water hose, see the backyard and all the rooms in the house. He said, "I want to see the color of Katherine's room and see the one that was supposed to be my bedroom."

All went well the next morning until he learned I was not going. "I can't go without you."

"Yes, you can, you are a big boy. You must learn to do things on your own and not always depend upon me. This is a very special day—the day belongs to you and your parents. It will be a happy day and I will be happy knowing that you are brave. I'll be here when you get back, and then I'll see you at seven tonight."

That evening a jovial David told me of what fun it had been to play with the hose, and how Katherine had screamed when he sprinkled her. The suit needed repairs, so it would be weeks before the next excursion. Although the home trip had been a great success, I couldn't see how the projected three trips per week could ever be managed.

On March 21, Arden Richardson reported at a CDP meeting on David's education. The kindergarten year was not progressing as well as expected. The teacher, who had worked with David in his home, felt strained and preferred not to teach David next year. Arden said, "David needs more than a homebound teacher, he needs group participation. If you don't make or allow some changes, he will take a very definite turn for the worse psychologically." The hospital attorney challenged her statements about the obligations of a school district. After she left, he referred to her as "a barracuda."

Upon returning to the hospital on April 18, David declared, "I'm just going to stay a short month and you are going to visit every night. I'm sad about coming back, I wanted to stay at home."

"I'm glad he feels sad coming back," I told Carol Ann. "It means he's a real member of the family."

I was with David when I was informed of my aunt's death. Acting very grown up, he tried to console me. "You said love never dies. Just the body dies—that 'you' always lives."

"That's right," I agreed. "But love is what makes us sad when someone we love dies."

I continued to be taken aback by the gaps in knowledge that David's world had imposed upon him. Referring to the cut apple logo on a Beatles record, David insisted that the picture was not a cross-section of a real apple—apples were either "applesauce or red." I brought him a green apple and cut it in half.

"You're right. I didn't believe you," he conceded. "Well, how do they make applesauce?"

"They cook and mash the apples." He proceeded to make applesauce by smashing the apple with his fist on the table. What a mess—apple all over the glove.

During every visit, David cried if I left before he went to sleep. "I'm afraid to go to sleep because of nightmares," he would complain. "There are holes in the bubble and I yell out loud, but no one hears me."

I had thought we had my leaving all worked out, but one night he pushed me to the limit. When I insisted firmly that I had to go, he wailed, "I understand, but you always have to go and do. Everybody does, and I can't!" Furious, he grabbed a green marker with the glove and it splattered all over my new sweater.

The next visit David announced, "I have made a decision. You are going to get married."

"Me, get married?"

"Yes, I got it all figured out. If you get married, your husband will have a car and live at your house. Then you can stay late every night until I'm asleep.

Then call your husband and tell him you are leaving. If you're not home in ten minutes, he can come out and look for you if your car broke."

"If I had a husband, he would object to my spending every evening with you."

"I don't see why."

"Tell you what, David, just take my word for it."

On May 5, Jackie and I received word from George Clayton, M.D., and the director of CRC: Our attendance at a communications meeting was "mandatory." We speculated—why? After the meeting, we still wondered—probably Brynn had complained about us.

The head nurse made the introductory remarks, "We are going to discuss David's behavior, in particular, his rudeness and angry behavior and consistency in discipline."

Brynn responded to Jackie's management tips with "Yes, but...." I did not bother to comment.

Nichols ruled, "I don't want people who have no meaningful relationship with David allowed in his room. If he doesn't react in a positive way, it gives us bad press." I chalked up another reason why I hated this man—appearance was far more important than David's distress. Jackie and I applauded Dr. Clayton's astute remark: "He needs peers, not adults."

The, nurses griped about David's outrageous, defiant behavior and verbal "zings." At that moment, I wished for a return of Louise and her group sessions.

Mary McKinney, Potts's assistant, who never had a problem with David, made a telling comment. "He doesn't act the same way with everyone."

Brynn, misunderstanding, agreed, "Yes, he does to each person what he knows will bother them the most."

The second excursion home in the space suit was scheduled for 8:45 an on Friday, May 12, 1978. I awoke Thursday midnight and realized that the space suit was probably too small by now, and this would be the last trip. I wanted the fun of going along. I lucked out; everyone on my CDP schedule canceled.

A few minutes after eight o'clock, I was in David's room. "I'm going with you."

Excited, he shouted to his mother, "I'm so happy! Mary is coming, too! She can ride in the van with us!"

"Hold it—I don't know where I'll ride, there may not be room in the van," I cautioned.

"I have to tell you one thing you have to do," David said, laughing. "Stay behind me, because I'm going to sprinkle and you will get wet if you don't stay behind."

"Water won't hurt me, but you can't sprinkle Jim's camera." While waiting to get in the suit, he had marked facial tics. He alternated between putting a puzzle together and huddling in my arms.

Once in the suit, he could not stand straight; he was too tall. Carol Ann was holding him during the wait to disconnect and she called me, "David wants both of us to hold him." He held her hand and my hand as he walked out of CRC.

In the basement, he again requested, "Please ride in the van with me."

"No, I am going to ride with your father in the other van."

They started the van and the air conditioning didn't work. After much commotion maintenance arrived, and Officer Roberts summoned me.

"David is getting anxious and his mother wants you in there," he said. I went in. It was hot, but David didn't complain, nor did he seem as uncomfortable as the rest of us. The air conditioner finally started.

As I left the van, he cried. Several people immediately yelled, in chorus, "Stay in here!" By this time, everyone was on edge and worried about the lost time. David wanted me to sit next to him. I said, "No, your mother should sit by you." After a hassle and compromise, I sat between him and the window, half on air, half on a side ridge.

David wasn't interested in looking at anything except the cameraman leaning out of the window to film us. I pointed out where I lived, "Just behind those trees, you can't see it, but it's right there."

"You mean back there?"

"Yes, right behind those trees."

"Mary, be sure to show me where you live on the way back."

At Carol Ann's urging, he waved at children in a school bus. She pointed out the hospital where Katherine had been born. He rocked or dozed most of the time.

The van parked on the street in front of David's home. He went down the ramp, but instead of going toward the house, he walked alongside the van and headed across the street saying, "I want to go in the backyard, not the front!" Ignoring all the shouts, he asserted adamantly, "No! No! I want to sprinkle in the back."

As he marched resolutely across the street, for the first time it became obvious to a large group of others that his perception of the physical world was different. Reluctantly and on faith alone, he turned around to go across the front lawn to the backyard, protesting all the way, "This is the wrong way!"

Once in the backyard, he was so excited to play with the hose again that he forgot that the yard was not where he expected to find it. He sprinkled Katherine, trees, and his dog. James de Leon called to me. They were holding a piece of Plexiglas in front of the camera and wanted to film David sprinkling the camera, but he refused to do so without my permission. I approached him from behind and yelled, "Sprinkle it, it's okay." Startled, he quickly turned, and I got soaked.

"I didn't mean to," he said. We both laughed.

The only item on the CDP curriculum was to walk completely around the house. We did. I carefully pointed out the back wall, the den window, the sidewall with the kitchen window, the front yard and the windows by his bubble, the other side with bedroom windows, and the back wall again. He exclaimed, "Gee, Mary, you're right, the house is a box and the backyard is where you said it was. You know everything."

He went into Katherine's room and pulled open a vanity drawer and threw things out. Unaccustomed to such brotherly trespass, she screamed. He also wanted to look at some of his records and bring one back.

When I told him it was time to go, he refused, but was obviously tired and did not resist vigorously. It was hot, ninety-two degrees, and the air conditioner once again did not work. He never complained but the rest of us were miserable. Security radioed. A ten-car pileup on Highway 45 necessitated a detour. David came to life, "A ten-car pileup, I want to see it!"

David had gone without drinking water or going to the bathroom for four hours. His wet hands stuck in the gloves. Katherine tried to help him pull his hands up out of the gloves, but he panicked and screamed. He had never before experienced heat or perspiration. Carol Ann and I had his hands in the suit arms when Brynn turned around and stridently yelled, "David, behave! All that's not necessary! Now shut up!"

Back at the hospital, David stood up to get out of the van and said, "Mary, hold one hand. Katherine holds the other."

That evening, I received an exuberant greeting. "Thank you for going with me—I had a good day because I spent so much time with you. I love you. Now I understand why it takes you only five minutes to get to the hospital from where you live.

"Tonight," he continued, "We are going to play a game—fish. Get in the gloves so I can tie a string to your finger. Now throw the string down into the playroom and say what you want hooked." This was the first time he had ever initiated a give-and-take game. The string broke, the knots slipped, but he didn't mind. Nothing altered his beaming happiness.

David's good mood was short-lived. The following Tuesday evening when I arrived, he was screaming at a CRC patient to get out. I apologized to the boy for David's behavior and said, "Bobby, please leave. I want to talk to David and see why he's so angry. I don't think it's you. You just happened to be here." Then, to David, "I'll listen to your side, but your cruelty is inexcusable!"

"I hate him, hate him, if I were out of here I'd smack him hard!" David cried. "I hate him. I don't want him in here. I don't want to look at him ever. He's blind! He's blind! He can't see anything! I can't stand it. It's too horrible for me to think about."

We discussed how awful life would be if you couldn't see. I again admonished, "Even though we feel terrible about or repulsed by a person's handicap, it does not give us the right to be cruel and hurt that human being."

The next day I caught a lizard and took it to him in a plastic bag. He became fascinated watching it turn green when on green paper and then brown again on the tabletop.

"Tape it to the bubble so I can really look at it. Is that the thing Renee says blows bubble gum?"

After the space suit walk around his family's home, David at least was willing to entertain the idea that his assumptions about the buildings across Fannin Street were incorrect. He conceded that Kelsey-Seybold did have four sides, but insisted the building had windows only in front. He had someone check the back of the clinic for windows. Unfortunately for the purposes of my teaching, the clinic had no windows in the back.

Despite my many attempts at explanation, the underpass at Fannin and Holcombe remained a mystery to David. From his vantage point, he could see cars on the one-lane surface frontage road continue at street level, while the cars in the center two lanes sank out of sight and seemingly vanished as they approached the underpass. Photographs taken by Jackie from all four sides failed to clarify its structure or function. I once asked him what he thought happened to all the disappearing cars, pointing out that "They have to come out someplace or they'd all pile up." He just looked blank.

His underpass confusion highlighted one of David's oddest misperceptions: that the ground's surface was like a sheet of paper, and there was simply "nothing" below its two-dimensional surface. David believed that trees and grass had no roots, and sand and dirt were not of earth or ground. He had a similar belief about the sky: that it was a blue bowl of a finite size.

Jackie undertook explaining trees and roots by bringing him a plant in a pot of soil. Using the big gloves, he pulled the plant up and plopped it back in the pot until the plant was spent, and all that remained was a pile of dirt. But the lesson with the flowerpot did not generalize to digging a hole in the ground.

When TV covered the funeral and grave site service of a prominent Houstonian, David asked, "Why the flowers? Where are the other coffins in the cemetery?"

"In graves."

"What's a grave? How do coffins get in graves?" Describing how a grave is dug and a casket is lowered into the hole to someone who doubts that anything exists beneath the ground's surface is difficult, and I was not sure

I was getting through. He listened intently as I groped for words, gestured, and drew pictures. Eventually I quit trying, and we played hide-and-go-seek.

The next visit, David declared, "Tonight we are going to have a funeral. I've got everything we need." He had little artificial flowers, a tiny box, and the flowerpot of dirt. I used ribbon and two pencils for a lowering device. We buried and dug up the casket time and time again. Perhaps, finally, he was grasping the concept of dirt below the ground's surface.

Perhaps because his life was governed by so many rules, David became obsessed with traffic signs. Jackie and I drew hundreds of them, taping them to the windows, the playroom, and the bubbles. He suggested that we look for new signs whenever we drove. I ordered a driver's license manual for him; it had pictures of every traffic sign in Texas.

We played and played "The Traffic Light Game." I was the signal, he the driver. He "drove" (scooting with hands and knees) back and forth in the playroom. I sat on a child's chair with my face in a glove so we could hear each other. He told me that red should be a loud, deep voice, yellow a low pitch, and green a high-pitched shriek. In the game, the driver doesn't heed the signal, but apologizes, gives preposterous excuses, and promises never, ever to do it again. After three law breaks, the signal calls the policeman.

In the fall David selected new wallpaper for the hospital room—white with blue sketches of trucks and traffic signs.

A TV program prompted dozens of questions on how cars were made—from the steel mill to the assembly line. How could red liquid metal become a car? My original major of mechanical engineering and years of work in a valve manufacturing plant came in handy. I rolled warm paraffin for "sheet metal" and poured hot wax in sand molds to cast the engine. With these crude parts, we constructed a car.

David grew tall so the crib isolator was made ten inches higher and a foot longer and the supply was enlarged. The new isolators were up at home, and when he got there on May 22, they weren't inflating properly. Mr. Langford solved the problem, but we were reaching the point where the bubbles couldn't be made larger and yet were functional. Bigger bubbles required more air pressure to stay inflated, more pressure than he could tolerate.

David's transfers to his home were becoming major productions. Brynn would be exhausted and in a foul mood. David would want to take everything home with him—the large blocks from the playroom and other things. I suggested, "Get another set of blocks to leave at home."

Brynn snapped, "There is no money to buy toys!" Arden and the teacher had told us that David was not making the expected progress in learning to read. Dr. Desmond brought in Nancy LaFevers, the CDP speech pathologist and education specialist. Nancy told me that the first time she met with the CDP team was an experience she would never forget:

"I was exposed for the first time to what David's life was like—what he could and could not have, the toileting, etc. I was horrified, not only at the restrictions of his situation but also at the staff. They seemed to take David's restrictions, his lack of control over his environment, as normal operating procedure, without sensitivity to his lack of privacy or needs as a child, a human being."

David's end-of-the-school-year reading achievement score was low. I argued against dyslexia, but was reminded that I had insisted he had perceptual problems. "Spatial, distance, and depth problems, yes," I said, "But not visual perception such as in a learning problem. He had a sight vocabulary of at least fifty words at age three. He finds titles and times in the TV Guide." What a flap. What if the press found out that the bubble boy had academic deficiencies?

Nancy contacted Sara Redd, a reading teacher and owner of a school for the learning disabled. Sara eagerly accepted the five-week assignment—an hour daily, four days per week for the nominal fee of $250 (the Women's Auxiliary picked up the tab). I knew Sara and knew David would like her. All agreed that David would be more accepting if I made the introduction.

After the first session, Sara reported, "He is not opposed to seeing me, he is opposed to my purpose for being with him. He is a very bright child with a wonderful vocabulary and simply a delight to be with."

She made a list of recommendations: small gloves, and so forth. "Sara," I said, "It's the same list I made four years ago."

Sara spent hours with him each day and concluded, "He reads, but doesn't know little words like 'the.' He's afraid to fail." I felt that this behavior was similar to his refusal to play games and stemmed from his feeling that he was already so defeated that he simply could not afford to lose. But as the days went by, his mastery improved; he was learning to read.

Arden came up with what I thought was a near-to-normal and practical schooling plan. He was to be registered in a regular first grade class at Lamar Elementary in Conroe. The teacher would be paid extra for going to his home early in the morning and then again after school. The teacher for the homebound would come for two hours a day (four days per week at the hospital, five days per week at home). Several children from the accelerated program would come to his house regularly to give him the sense of being part of a class. This system was instituted, and worked fairly well.

The older David grew, the more aware he was becoming of just how unique his predicament was. At age six he began saying, "Why me? Why me? Why me in this bubble? Why me and the space suit? Why me? Why me? Why do I have to live this way? Why am I in this? Give me answers! Tell me why!" After one of these outbursts, I held him tightly for a long time, saying nothing.

"You can't tell me why. No one can tell me why I have to be in here. So what is the answer?"

"Love, I don't have the power or knowledge to answer your questions. I don't know of anybody who does."

"I know if you could help me or answer, you would. Who could help me?"

"Someday, research will find an answer, but that time is probably far in the future. I understand how you feel. Your pain is my pain. We can't change or fix things. What we can do is change how we deal with things and that's what we're going to do. The important thing is how we deal with this whole predicament."

"I'm glad we've had this talk," said David, brightening somewhat. "Now, let's play hide-and-go-seek."

The next day I ate lunch with him while his mother looked at films of David. When she came in, she said somberly, "My son looks so sad in most of the pictures."

8.

THE SEVEN-YEAR-OLD PLAYWRIGHT

"I wish the anger would go away. Remember our angry games? How many years did we play them?"

"Two, maybe three. We started right around your seventh birthday." "Yeah, I remember the first one: 'Mary Gets Mugged.'"

When David returned to the hospital on July 5, 1978, he openly discussed his anger. He equated loss of control and anger with going crazy. "Why am I so angry all the time? Why am I angry with people? Why am I so angry at things that never did anything to me? What do other boys do when they get angry like this?"

"They run outside, slam the door, and ride their bicycles, or do something until the anger is gone," I explained. "They discharge anger in a physical way that doesn't get them in trouble. You don't have any opportunity or way to do that. The best you can do is run races on a six-foot track."

"Whatever I do depends on what somebody decides I do. Why school? Why did you make me learn to read? What good will it do? I won't ever be able to do anything anyway, so why? You tell me why!"

"I can't say why, but it's a waste of energy to blame or curse. It doesn't do any good. It makes things worse."

"Sometimes I get so angry, I say or do something awful—then I'm sorry and feel bad, and everybody gets mad at me. I think I'm going crazy."

"Trouble is, you hold it all in until you explode." "Why?"

"I'm not sure I can explain. If someone lives with an ever-present danger, it inevitably leads to anger. So in part, your anger comes from your constant and sensible fear of germs. The other part is that everyone needs to have some control over their world so they can be competent and learn to grow up, be self-sufficient. When something stops you or gets in your way of becoming independent, it just naturally leads to frustration and anger. So often I've heard you say, 'I can't do it by myself. If I could figure out a way to do it myself, I would.' When you totally depend on people, you dare not show anger; you hold it in and hide it. You don't want others to be angry with you, retaliate, or think you're an awful person. Problem is, if you hold it in all the time, you have so much anger inside that the least little thing upsets you. You don't think, you just explode."

"I know what you're getting at, but—"

"I know getting so angry and losing control is scary, but it doesn't mean you're going crazy. I don't like using the slang word crazy, but anyway, crazy people have imaginary problems and never worry about going crazy. Your problems are real and you worry. So you are not crazy."

"Okay, Miss Reality."

"You don't realize it, but you're far more responsible and capable than most boys your age. I don't know any other kid who could do all the things you must do. You are smart."

"I was born with a good brain—right?"

"Right, and so was I, and we're going to start using them now. We can't change the fact that you live in isolation, but we can learn to deal with your situation better. If all you do is awfulize, you'll always be upset and miserable. I'm going to make a cup of tea and when I return, I want my usual happy greeting—big smile and head bump. We are going to start the whole evening over and take each day one at a time."

As I went for my tea, I worried. I had thought David would be at least nine years old before we had this conversation. Here he was," barely seven, and already awash in rage at the restrictions in his life. What would happen when he was nine or twelve and fully cognitive of the bleakness of his future as an adult? No matter how much love and attention his parents gave, or how much Jackie and I worked to enhance his self-esteem, he was going to feel more and more alienated and bitter. With everything in his life situation ruinous, I knew he could not help but doubt his worth. No freedom. No choices. No ways to move on and find a goal, anticipate the future, or acquire a sense of belonging. He could not do chores or be an active, responsible family member, let alone be a part of a peer group.

Anger—what it was and what to do about it—was to become one of our most frequent topics of conversation.

Perhaps to convince himself that his anger was not so unique, David often asked me to tell him about the times in my life when I was most angry. He then turned my responses into plays.

For example, I told him about my mugging: two men had knocked me down, dragged me across the parking lot, but had given up trying to shove me in a car. Store security, anxious to get bloody me out of the sight of Christmas shoppers, had ushered me into an office and called the police. The policeman had asked ridiculous questions.

In David's improvised play, he was the policeman; I was myself.

Policeman: Name please.

Mary: Mary Ada Murphy.

Policeman: Age please.

Mary: What difference does my age make?

Policeman: It says here I have to ask how old you are.

Mary: Over twenty.

Policeman: Are you married?

Mary: What does my marital status have to do with this? Let me give you the first three numbers of the license plate.

Policeman: No, it says here I have to ask if you're married.

Mary: I refuse to answer.

Policeman: Type of crime? We can't call this robbery, they didn't steal anything. It isn't murder, you're still alive.

Mary: How about assault?

Policeman: Yeah, that's good—assault.

At his home, David asked his father to watch us perform the plays. His father laughed hysterically and considered "The Tire Salesman" the most hilarious. It was based on a premise stated by David: "If a person is a really good salesman, he can sell square tires."

The story begins with a customer saying he needs a size XYZ tire. The salesman says he doesn't have that size in a round tire, but has it in a square tire that works even better. The salesman has a reply for each of the customer's "yes, buts" and insists that the only important thing about buying a new tire is that the inner rim that fits on the car be round; it doesn't matter if the outside is square.

David Sr. said, "Son, you are so persuasive you could sell me an XYZ square tire."

David's fascination with the emotion of anger continued the rest of his life. When he was ten, he called me from his home and excitedly exclaimed, "Mary, Mary, you'll never guess what happened! I was looking out of the window, and a car stopped at the intersection. After a while, a teenager got out and opened the hood and did something, then he got back in the car, and then he got back out and looked at the engine, and then he slapped the hood down, and got on top of it and kicked the windshield until it broke! Then he walked away."

"What happened to the car?"

"He just left it and then there was a man, I think it was his dad, who came in a pickup truck, and they pulled it away. It was just like our angry games. It didn't do him any good to get angry, he only broke his car more."

One reason anger fascinated, and frightened, David so much was that he never experienced anyone's but his own—he had no normal experience in everyday life situations. Jackie described his interaction with the classmates who came to his house as "artificial and contrived, with a select group well prepared for the circumstances. Normal groups are set up by the children themselves, not adults." The layout of his parents' house did not allow David to see social interaction—because his isolator filled the living-dining room, the family and guests usually spent time in the den. Also, his mother protected him from anything unpleasant. As a result, he never understood arguments.

"Did you get a divorce because of arguments?" he once asked me.

"No."

"Well, my parents had an argument, and I'm worried that they might get a divorce. They never, ever had an argument before, just this one."

"If two people care for each other and live together, it's impossible to not have disagreements and arguments. Any truly intimate love relationship has both good and bad times."

"So you are saying I should be worried if they never had an argument. Arguments are just part of living." "You got it."

"Why did you get a divorce?"

"I didn't expect that one. Probably because there was nothing left between my husband and me, we didn't even bother to argue."

The patients on CRC provided David few opportunities to interact with peers. Most of the children suffered chronic or debilitating diseases. David liked a pretty girl his age with a rare metabolic disorder called argininemia. Gracie, severely retarded, spoke in single words and comprehended only simple phrases. He said, "You have to talk very carefully to Gracie." He delighted in teaching her a new word and didn't mind that Potts was very fond of her.

Another girl, five years older than David, had horrific endocrine problems, both legs had been amputated and she had no hair, but she was very bright and sociable. David kept asking me questions about her prosthesis that I couldn't answer. I suggested he invite her in. He did. She spontaneously explained her medical condition and how the prosthesis worked.

Though not sheltered in the physical sense as David was, these children also led somewhat sheltered lives. They did not provide David with a chance to explore the intricacies of anger.

David informed me, "Dr. Feigin is the big boss, and you know what? Since he came and goes to the CDP meetings, you got some authority around this place." Jackie expressed her thoughts: "Although Dr. Feigin isn't always here, I always feel his presence and support. Also, I think part of that feeling is because David has a very clear picture of where Dr. Feigin is in the hierarchy. David's fond of saying, 'I know where the power is in the hospital—it's Dr. Feigin.'"

David asked me to explain why the doctors and I wore Baylor badges and the nurses and Jackie wore hospital ones. I explained the affiliation between Baylor and TCH, "The medical school faculty directly supervises the clinical services in the hospital. All the chiefs of services and their assistants are Baylor professors." He studied the flow chart I drew and was able to understand where everyone stood in relation to Baylor and hospital administration.

"Dr. Feigin really is the boss. I was right."

A welcome change came two weeks before David's seventh birthday. On September 11, 1978, William Shearer, M.D., Ph.D., recently appointed professor of Pediatrics, Microbiology, and Immunology, was named David's attending physician. Dr. Shearer appeared very serious and formal; I couldn't imagine his ever having been a little boy. A disciplined scientist, compassionate pediatrician, and devout Roman Catholic, he held rigid authoritative rules for child rearing. In no way did David fit this model. Jackie considered Dr. Shearer too aloof and somberly austere to relate to comfortably. I learned to know him when we discussed, at length, David's history.

Jackie, Dr. Desmond, and I were pleased with Dr. Shearer's methodical physician-patient approach and plan of a thorough study of David's immunological status, though his remoteness surprised the usually effervescent Carol Ann. After chatting with him for a few minutes before a CDP meeting and getting no response, she stopped mid-sentence, laughed, and said, "I'm wasting my time flirting with you, aren't I?" He blushed, Jackie and I laughed.

Dr. Shearer operated under three premises: the first, that David was a patient, not an exhibit. Under no circumstance would he introduce a curiosity seeker to David. He never veered from this. He said no to the Crown Prince of Iran.

He did not enjoy such success with his second premise, that David, as a patient and a child, would do as he was told. David shattered that illusion.

This third premise was that he would not make the mistake of the original doctors and become personally involved with David and his family. He didn't count on David's personality and strength of character. In time, he came to respect, admire, and even love this extraordinary boy.

9.

LOOKING OUT FROM THE ISOLATOR

"*Look at that view; it's nothing,*" *David said, staring at the brick wall that faced our window.* "*How long would it take to construct a model of that? How would you start?*"

"*Less than an hour. A box could be the court, and a piece of cardboard the brick wall. We could cut a hole in the box for this window, draw the other windows on the inside of the box, draw bricks on the wall, and tape it up.*"

"*Gee, is that all? It took us months to build the model of Fannin Street.*"

"*You had to keep plucking new green trees from the bushes.*"

We had duplicated everything David could see—buildings, lampposts, and parking lot—and mounted it on a large piece of cardboard. He never pitched a tantrum over this project because I made everything to his specifications. He firmly believed the distant Shamrock Hilton Hotel was the smallest building when, in reality, it was the largest. He held to his trust in appearance, so I made it the smallest.

From the windows, which faced west, David saw the doctors' parking lot, a two-story hospital annex, a traffic artery and, across the street, a variety of buildings. Directly opposite was a one-story bank, to his left a fourteen-story Holiday Inn, and to the right a five-story medical clinic, Kelsey-Seybold. He could see the front as well as the roof of the bank and two sides of both the clinic and the Holiday Inn. To his left, a block away, he could see the

Holcombe-Fannin and Interfirst Bank buildings and the front of the more distant Shamrock Hilton Hotel.

Many times I wished for a street perpendicular to Fannin and David's hospital window so he could view cars getting smaller as they drove away and larger as they approached. Although his home in Conroe was at an intersection, and his isolator provided him a clear view out of the living room's picture window, the house across the street blocked a distant view.

The Interfirst Bank and the Shamrock Hilton both have approximately sixteen stories. The Shamrock, however, is a much larger building in terms of square feet. It was impossible to convince him that the hotel was the larger of the two structures and appeared smaller only due to the effect of distance. He never understood size constancy—that we attribute the actual size of a distant object to the associations it represents in our minds, rather than how it actually looks. David understood that a row of windows represented a floor, and after counting the stories in each building, he reluctantly agreed they were the same height, but he could not comprehend the more complex issue of square footage or the amount of ground covered by the Shamrock Hilton.

Later, when he was eleven, a weather circumstance, fog, helped to give David a vague precept of distance. On a foggy night, when the Holiday Inn lights were brighter than the Interfirst Bank's, and the more distant Shamrock Hilton's lights were barely visible, he said that one of my many demonstrations of size constancy now made sense: "I think I understand what you were trying to get at when you walked away holding the little flashlight."

Jackie and I concluded from observing David's perceptual development for years that neither looking at buildings, photographs, and television, nor the use of the power of cognition, can substitute for experience. Phenomena must be experienced to be learned.

Few people realized that David's precepts did not agree with objective reality because David took care to hide his mistakes. He frankly discussed the discrepancy between his observations or assumptions and other descriptions of the physical world with Jackie and me, as well as his father, because, having lost trust in his own fallible perception, he needed to check out reality with us. But with others, he never did so. In a conversation, he feared making a blunder and appearing "stupid." Therefore, he cautiously listened for cues so he could monitor himself and quickly cover errors.

For example, Nancy LaFevers, the speech therapist, once brought an eleven-year-old girl to visit. Andrea Ambroze, who loved horses, brought sketches—racehorses, quarter horses, farm horses. David showed interest in the pictures because she had drawn them. Looking at a racing sulky he said, "Oh, that's the thing that makes the horse go."

Andrea looked confused. He shot me a quick glance, I indicated no.

He laughed, "I had you going there, didn't I? You really believed I thought the cart made the horse go."

Later, Nancy commented on this, her first meeting with David: "I reeled with emotion upon visiting David in his bubble. The helplessness of his circumstance—the restrictions of his environment on his movement through and interactions with the world—was overwhelming!

David had binoculars outside the bubble, but the PVC distorted his view. I ordered a cardboard telescope. When it arrived, I struggled, listened to David's advice, but couldn't assemble it. He suggested Mr. Langford could do it.

"You're right, I'll put it back in the box. You call him in the morning." Mr. Langford came to my office, "This is junk. Why didn't you buy the kid a decent one?"

"That junk is the only telescope in the world free of lubricant.

He assembled it, but it didn't have enough power for David to really see things from the time I first worked with David, I made periodic checks of the latest journals and collected hundreds of articles on visual-spatial perception but found only three that had relevance to David's case. Since Jackie's and my roles with David were not public knowledge, we were never approached by researchers, and our intimacy with David precluded our ever placing him into a situation of experimental study. I did, however, discuss my observations with several psychologists. One, Joseph Pagan, III, Ph.D., of Case Western, showed interest. He encouraged me to keep notes and to contact the renowned visual perception theorist, James Gibson, Ph.D. I phoned Dr. Gibson and he made arrangements for me to read an advance copy of his latest work, *The Ecological Approach to Visual Perception*. He assured me his book would clear up all my questions. His theory that visual perception is direct and does not require interpretation or experience did not agree with my observations of David. David's description of his world as flat silhouettes was the exact opposite of Gibson's position: "No one ever saw the world as a flat patchwork of colors... The notion of a patchwork of colors comes from the art of painting, not from any unbiased description of visual perception."

Jackie and I thought the theory of famed cognitive theorist Jean Piaget—that realty is constructed out of experience—held the most promise in understanding David's perceptual development. In Piagetian terms, David never developed beyond the sensory-motor stage in knowing spatial concepts.

In *The Mechanisms of Perception,* Piaget's "oyster and rock" can be seen as analogous to David and his bubble:

"If we passed our lives fixed to a solid object, as do oysters to a rock, and were deprived of movement and manipulations... size constancy would probably not develop."

Although many would probably disagree, Jackie and I were convinced that David's limited visual perception was due not only to deprivation, but also to egocentrism; he was never able to distinguish between other's precepts and his own. Before being in the space suit, David proclaimed that there were only four places in the hospital: CRC, Jackie's office, the garage, and CDP. While on the elevator with him in the space suit, we stopped on each floor and opened the door. He counted, checked the numbers, and conceded that there were seven floors.

David's egocentric perception interfered with his TV watching. Despite repeated encouragement from Jackie and me, his interest in the world through travel documentaries remained minimal.

He preferred stories enacted in one room. He liked the characters on "*Little House on the Prairie,*" but he needed an interpreter when the action moved outside. "The wagon disappeared, what happened?" It had gone over a hill.

I stood looking at David, so ill, so frail, and was consumed with anger, thinking, Why couldn't he have been out of the bubble a few weeks earlier so he could have been wheeled around the hospital and down to the parking lot?

"Remember the dollhouse in the Christmas catalogue?" he asked. "How can I forget? You have mentioned it every day since before the holidays. You should have let me buy it. I wanted it, really, but what would people say? A twelve-year-old boy with a dollhouse."

"Remember when we made the two-story house? "Sure, that was three or four years ago, but you've referred to it several times lately."

I had glued two shoeboxes together and made a picket railing around the top. That rain would pour through the hole in the roof he wanted for viewing the stairs never occurred to him, and I certainly didn't mention it. The important thing was to be sure one could see the stars from the porch.

I wondered, what does the dollhouse represent to him? What is his fantasy? Is he asking, is this a real home? Is this what I missed? Is this living in the world?

We cried and reached out to each other. We couldn't embrace—the tubes in his chest. We dared not bump heads. We held hands. He whispered, "Mary, your problem is you care too much."

10.

SEVEN YEARS IN THE BUBBLE

"Donna Aldridge called; she is sad I'm so sick." "I know, she's been keeping in close touch."

"Remember when she started as my nurse?"

"Yes, you were seven. She began in January 1979 so she would learn how to do everything before Brynn left in June."

"Yeah, they worked at preparing me for Brynn's leaving. It was sad that she had to go with her husband to a city where she didn't know anybody. My mother didn't want her to leave. They were good friends—talk, talk, all the time."

In April of 1979, joyous excitement—the newly built crib had fitted gloves for David. At seven-and-a-half years of age, a new world opened for him.

Even though the isolator had proved a constant source of frustration, I had never considered the PVC a barrier to our intimacy. Yet, the first time I was with him when he had his hands in the fitted gloves was memorable—true, rare intimacy. The small gloves, thinner plastic than the big ones, allowed for more tactile sensation and an almost instant feeling of warmth.

David ordered me to sit on the stool and roll up close. He placed both hands on top of my head and ran his fingers through my hair, then lovingly caressed my face before moving his hands down my neck, across my shoulders, and down my arms; at last, grasping my hands, he locked eyes and smiled—an incredulous, lingering smile. Carol Ann described a similar experience.

David could do everything in the fitted gloves—color with markers, operate the record player and the TV remote control, work on our construction projects, and even organize my purse. The first thing he checked for was the American Express card. "You should never leave home without it," he cautioned.

He hid my keys by sliding them between the crib floor and the tabletop. He laughed and laughed. "I got you, really got you. You can't leave. Tell you what, if in the morning you can't button your blouse in the back, you come up here and drink your coffee while I button." In general, he was in a good mood during this period, but his intense thumb sucking and simultaneous nose rubbing irritated the staff.

Along with the gloves, his world was opening in other ways. First, the "telephone booth" transport was ordered. As it had for the other bubbles, Standard Safety Equipment, in Illinois, furnished the PVC shell. The nurses cut the holes and placed gloves in the port rings. After completion, they filled the bubble with Freon to detect leaks, rinsed with water, and sterilized with peracetic acid. The transport was mounted on plywood, which fit in a foot-high metal wagon built at the hospital, and connected to the playroom.

David was to enter the new transport bubble on Monday, May 28, 1979. Sunday night he cheerfully quipped, "Hello, best friend. Best friend, who knows how to make a friend, who knows how to let people go to sleep. Best friend, who lets me make a lovely mess. Best friend, you will be here in the morning when I get in the transport to go home, won't you?"

The next morning, excited and in a good humor, he requested, "Mary, would you please come down here by the sleeve to the transport?" I did, he crawled in, stood up alongside me, and enthusiastically exclaimed, "This is my favorite bubble!"

He scampered back into the playroom and returned with an intricate control panel made of Lego toy bricks. He taped it to the inside of the transport, asserting, "Now we really have our space ship. Get the little chair you sit on when you talk through the glove and sit beside me. I'm rescuing you from the moon." And so we were off on a wondrous trip in outer space.

James de Leon came in saying, "This will make a great shot."

David took the panel down. "Please... It's private between Mary and me."

Six weeks later, back at the hospital, David, cuddled in my gloved arms, declared, "Mary, you could not deny me anything."

"Well, I'm not sure I'd go that far. What do you want?" "Oh, nothing. When you are alone, are you lonely?" "What are you trying to say or ask for?"

"Oh, nothing, really nothing."

Five days later he finally came out with it, "Is it my imagination or did you one time show me goldfish?"

"Yes."

He queried, "Well, could you do it again?" "Sure, Mildred still has a goldfish; I'll get it."

After watching the fish for a long time and asking, "Is it real, really?" Just then the fish poo-pooed. "It IS real! Would you please get two real ones for me? Do you think we would be in trouble?"

Actually, I had often thought of getting him fish because my son had enjoyed aquariums, but a newspaper headline, "David Thrives in His Fishbowl," had made me shun them because the association bothered me.

But since, as David said, I could not deny him anything, on Saturday, August 11, 1979, I took him two goldfish. "Are they mine, really mine?" he asked.

I forewarned him that the fish might die, and, as I had figured, they lived only a few weeks. Actually, it was amazing they survived that long, because David was forever reaching his gloved hands into the bowl to rearrange the rocks, and he always overfed them. He was sad that they died, but not inconsolable.

I then bought two guppies. Early the next morning, a Sunday, the phone woke me. A shrill voice I didn't immediately recognize kept saying, "Guess what? Mary, guess what?"

"I don't know; tell me."

"The girl fish had babies!"

"How many?"

"Too numerous to count. Come quick!"

From then on, we usually had at least three fish bowls: one for the baby guppies, one for the parents, and one for a male beta that David's grandmother had purchased for him. Then the beta needed a "wife," so that meant a fourth bowl. I was less than enthusiastic about cleaning the fish bowls and Carol Ann shared my feelings, but the fish provided hours of entertainment, and for long periods David watched them swim. He told Jackie, "I just love to watch my fish." He ordered different colored rocks, a treasure chest, houses, and plants.

The guppies were prolific—many new babies. In the meantime, the male Beta built one bubble nest after another for the female's eggs. Breeding betas proved too complicated for us. David, confused by the two means of reproduction, eggs and live birth, ordered, "Buy a book on fish reproduction."

This request had nothing to do with sex; he was strictly interested in reproduction. I read several chapters and he said, "That's enough." After serious meditation, he concluded, "Now, I understand why there has to be a male."

David was not able to reach the wall-mounted phone by the crib; therefore someone had to press the receiver against the bubble so he could listen and talk. A whole new world opened for him when he realized that with the fitted gloves in the transport he could operate, without assistance, the phone that sat on the floor. He misdialed when calling his friend Shawn who often visited David at his home in Conroe. What fun—getting a wrong number!

He then dialed numbers at random to talk to strangers. He said, "This is David, the Boy in the Bubble." Not believing him, they laughed but usually talked.

Other good things happened that summer. Potts found new, sterile foods—soup, spaghetti, chocolate milkshakes, and baked apples. Donna lined the potty with plastic bags instead of diapers. Good riddance! Visitors seeing the stacks of diapers and baby bottles had to wonder! He gained some privacy and control; from the transport he could open and close the red drape across the hall door. Plans were made to put curtains in the playroom.

On September 5, 1979, the Baylor photographers filmed David at home for his eighth birthday press releases. Distraught, he questioned Donna, "Why does this have to be done? Do you know how it feels to have all this done? What do they want from me? What are they after? I don't want to see this film show up on TV because I don't want to see myself on TV again. This can't go on every September. Next year I'm not going to do this! It's going to take weeks to get the playroom panel replaced." (The camera lights had melted the Plexiglas.)

After awhile he asked, "Donna, do you know what it is like to have too many people who love you? Too many people come to your house?" She tried to explain that she did but he argued, "You don't understand, I don't understand, and neither does Mom."

Later that month, when David returned to the hospital, Kaylen Fry of Baylor public relations phoned to ask me to participate in the upcoming press conference because I could provide firsthand anecdotes. I informed Kaylen that I didn't have the authority to say yes. She would have to clear it with Dr. Desmond. I warned, "My role has never been made public and I'm to maintain low visibility."

Within a few minutes, Dr. Desmond indignantly charged into my office. "I will not allow you to take part in the press conference. Reporters are vicious. They will tear you to shreds—eat you alive. I have to stop this. I'm going to tell Dr. Feigin that you are not capable of handling the press."

Kaylen phoned, "I'm sorry—you would have been good, but I understand Dr. Desmond's position. She is responsible for your actions and whatever you say."

At the press conference, Dr. Desmond spoke of David's "large vocabulary" and "blossoming social skills."

David had requested that only Mom and the CRC staff attend his hospital birthday party, but many others came. According to Donna, he could barely be polite and then cried, "I'm not enjoying this. The whole staff knew everything about the party, and I didn't and don't now."

The party was in another room. Everyone ate cake and ice cream except him.

David went home on September 19 and enjoyed the celebration of his eighth birthday. He watched the TV coverage with his parents and commented, "Hey, there's Dr. Shearer!" He questioned, "Mom, what do they mean by 'oldest surviving'? "

"Some children whose body can't fight germs aren't protected in a bubble and get very ill." He asked no more questions.

My mother and I visited David the day after the party.

To Aunt Patty's question of how much longer we could all go on, I replied, "Not long. Not long at all."

More problems: The government banned the sale of Quickspray, which was used to patch the PVC. Polykleen, used to take the "cloud" off the PVC, was dangerous.

Concerns were raised that the substances used to sterilize items given to David were toxic. OSHA, TCH Safety Committee, and Baylor Biomedical Department set out rules. Now the nurses had to wear masks and heavy acid resistant gloves and body garments when spraying items into the bubble. David worried about the fact that he encountered the stuff unprotected. I stated, truthfully, that the biggest danger to the nurses was to unborn babies they might be carrying. That seemed to satisfy him.

David's growing up necessitated heightening the crib isolator so he could stand straight. Having his head touch the top accentuated his poor posture. The taller bubble did not remain taut, and the sagging caused creases and eventual cracks. When the crib was thirty-six-inches high, the system was sleek and streamlined. Now it was a scary-built, decrepit contraption with patches everywhere and yards and yards of fiberglass tape wrapped around and around the weak spots at the ports and air nozzles. The implications of David's loss of trust in the isolation system and brittle emotional state were staggering. His feelings of helplessness were equaled only by Jackie's and mine.

As David's fame grew, Donna had more and more problems with visitors. Some had nothing to do with TCH; others were employees. People believed they had a right to come in and look at the "curiosity." The CDP team discussed the need for a firm policy from public relations.

Another incident brought this problem to a head. President Carter's daughter, Amy, invited David to the White House. This called for worry among the physicians and grave but colorful discussions—What about the publicity? How do you say no to the daughter of the President of the United States? A trip to the White House would have been virtually impossible. No one—not the President nor the public—understood the severe limitations of David's world. We respectfully had to decline.

Meanwhile, David wanted shoes and *Star Wars* toys for Christmas. Donna, after a struggle, got the shoes sterilized, but I never saw him wear them— he stayed with socks on.

On December 19, with relief, Jackie and I bid him off for home. Surely everything would be better after the holidays. We were wrong. The new year started with a power failure in the night. Before David's parents could put stoppers on the outlets, the bubble had collapsed—a terrifying experience for him.

When he went home before Christmas, he weighed fifty-two pounds. When he returned in January 1980, he had lost three and a half pounds. "It's just been too much of a hassle to eat," he said.

11.

AGE EIGHT—THE BEGINNING OF THE END

"I'm remembering Bill's paintings. It would be nice to see them—to have Eternity in here," David said.

"No way could we get an oil canvas sterile and in this room. I could bring Eternity to the door and let you see it."

"No. It's all right. I know it exactly. Remember—you didn't see the important things. I had to show you."

The summer before David's eighth birthday had actually marked the beginning of the end. Painfully aware of being different and not belonging to a peer group, he said, "Let's face it—what do I have in common with kids my age? Nothing."

The absence of goals to provide a reason for being and doing, together with his haunting dread of being deserted, compounded his anguish and feelings of alienation. He struggled to maintain control over his emotions as he tried to find an answer to his existence and what lay beyond death.

During the May 1979 hospital stay, David repeatedly made vague comments concerning death and trust, but would not further disclose his troubled thoughts. Two events deeply disturbed him: A dragonfly, caught in a spider web, hung dead outside the window. Hysterical, he demanded it be removed and refused to eat as long as it was there. Next, Jackie's dog Duffy died; he mourned as much or more than Jackie.

Carol Ann had taken pains to shield David from the knowledge of the death of his older brother. One Saturday evening, he stated, "No one in my family ever died. Lots of your family died—your dad, Renee's mother, and your dogs, but no one in my family dies."

"No, you're wrong," I told him. "People die in all families, grandparents and great-grandparents. It's a cycle, one generation dies and another is born."

"No, not in my family." Death and trust were becoming two of his most frequent topics; he quickly shifted the conversation to the latter: "People can't be trusted. Why do people say one thing and do another? Even their faces say something different from their words."

"You know, I believe trust is important and basic to every relationship. I prefer to believe that people can be trusted, I'm not as cynical and skeptical as you."

"Did you see the new patient? She was born premature and can't eat. I'm not like her. I was born perfect."

For my dissertation, I was comparing the stress of families with a handicapped child two to eight years of age, with that of families with intact children. David, in on every step of the study, worried about my control group.

"It's easy to get kids with a problem. This hospital is full of them, but I don't know where you will find a hundred healthy kids."

Wednesday evening, Kurt, an eight-year-old boy who was being treated for short stature, came into David's room and we engaged in a three-way conversation. Kurt brought in a toddler barn toy: push a button and out pops a blue lamb, a white hen sitting on a nest, a yellow duck, a pink pig, or a spotted cow.

Much to my surprise, David misnamed the chicken, pig, and lamb. I thought, "This is unbelievable. Ten minutes ago we were discussing a doctoral dissertation, and now he doesn't know the difference between a lamb and a pig."

David kept the barn, and it became the inspiration for a series of David-produced plays that left me very disturbed about his mental state. Saturday night David said, "Mary, tell you what, pretend these animals are your baby mice. I am putting them in the barn, and then you can never touch them again. You can see them, but not touch. Mary, these are your baby mice and I'm going to put them in the barn, and you can never ever touch them again and you must be sad. Now, pretend you are very sad and cry."

Each time he ordered, "Now you must be very, very sad!" Then, again, "Now this time be really, very, very, very sad, and do a good cry because you can never touch your babies again."

We had worked out other problems through playacting so I decided to continue, although I was uncomfortable. After a while I said, "It is sad for me that you are in the bubble, and I know it's sad for your mother and sad for you."

While David often expressed dismay about his captivity, he also frequently insisted, perhaps in an attempt to convince himself, that he was perfectly content. He did so now. "Oh, no, not me. I am happy in the bubble," he retorted. "Out there you all have to worry about germs, and I don't. And, what's more, you have to worry about insects, and I don't. See, I can stand here and watch a mosquito fly by and not worry that it will bite me."

The next evening David continued with the gruesome plays. He decided after I cried and was sad he would kill my baby mice with a "special" gas capsule or by burning the barn. Each time he killed the mice, I was to be sadder and cry harder. He embellished more and more after I knew that I couldn't touch my babies any more, I was to leave the room for a little bit, come back, and discover them dead.

The next evening, he stated, "I have a new play. I am the wife, you are the husband. You come home from work happy and smiling and say hello and all that stuff. We're real happy. Then you're supposed to ask about your baby mice and insist on seeing them. Now go outside and come back in smiling."

"Hello, husband. How are you? You look happy." "Oh, yes, I'm happy. How are my babies?"

"Oh, they're all right. They are in the other room." "I want to see my babies right now."

"No, they're asleep. Just leave them alone."

He laid out the rest of the script: go into the room, find the babies dead, and be angry because the wife didn't take the right kind of care of them. The wife (with a silly grin and high-pitched voice) was to say that she gassed them, burned them, drowned them, poisoned them, or shot them.

In another version, "When you find the babies dead, say, 'You didn't take care of my babies. You didn't feed them, you didn't give them water, you put them in a plastic bag with no blowers. You are a poor wife and mother!' "

Playing the wife, David responded: "Oh, no, no. I fed them. I gave them water, and I gave them plenty of oxygen. I didn't neglect them at all. I took good care of them. I killed them because I hated them. I hated 'em, I hated 'em, I hated 'em! (Taken aback at being carried away with anger he drew himself together.) No, I didn't hate them at all. I loved them."

In his final script, "I'll hold my babies like this and dump them in the ocean so they drown; but before I drop them in the ocean, I'll tie a piece of meat on their backs so the sharks will be sure to eat them."

Upset with myself for letting him go too far, I was relieved when he smiled and abruptly changed the subject.

"Now tell me about those kids you've seen—those ones that weren't born perfect. But I had to be told, before I was born, that I was going to be put in a bubble when I was born."

"You were told?"

"Sure. Otherwise, if I had been born and wound up in a bubble and didn't know it ahead of time, I would have gone bananas. So I knew all about it."

"Who told you and how?"

"This is the way it was: First there was a little egg that went down the passage. It went down first, and it told me I would have to be in a bubble when I was born."

"You mean this little egg went down the passage first and told you the future?"

"Yes, before I was born there was this little egg, and it met with this other little thing, and it went *Wham!* and it was born before I was born. He told me I would be in a bubble."

At this point, I thought: I'm a basket case.

His jolly mood continued. "We're going to take off to Mars and see the beautiful moon and stars. All the women on earth will be destroyed. I'm taking you with me. I'll always keep you safe. You're my copilot."

David's interest in space and astronomy went beyond our flying around. He asked Jackie for a moon globe and stated, "If they're going to explore outer space, they will have to send a pregnant girl so the baby can live to be old enough to get to the faraway planets."

On Monday, May 28, as we wheeled David down the hall to go home in the new transport, he instructed, "Hurry and get your research paper going so mother can fill out one of those questionnaires before my eighth birthday. Remember, I am a control. I was born perfect."

After a stay at home, David returned to the hospital on July 12, 1979. When I arrived at quarter past seven that evening, he was agitated, rocking and thumb sucking.

"Well, after one thousand years you get here. Why haven't you ever mentioned my brother?"

"No reason, I never saw him."

"I'm angry because my parents never discussed my brother with me before now."

Still, he seemed to get over his anger quickly this time. I knew talk of his brother was over when he said, "Let's get our exercises over with so we can play." As we jumped rope he yelled, "You might as well give up; you're never gonna get the hang of jumping. Let's do sit-ups."

While David was home in September for his eighth birthday, Dr. Shearer told me he had completed the tests on David's immune system and a cure was probably at least ten years away. I said, "We'll never make it. If I give one thought to adolescence, I won't make it through the day, today." He asked if I thought anyone had ever talked honestly with David's parents about the realities and the future.

"No," I replied. "They have been encouraged to wait for the miracle that is just around the corner."

He discussed the limited treatment protocols available—fetal thymus or liver transplants or incompatible bone marrow. I said, "I know the horror of graft-versus-host disease from the bone marrow transplants Dr. Montgomery did here on CRC. I can't bear to think of that for David—rotting away."

We then discussed another patient, a severely brain-damaged child on life-support systems that I had to evaluate. My view: "Death would be a luxury for this child. Why prolong life to no avail? If she survives, she will never be aware of anything, except maybe pain."

He agreed. "Hospitals have become places to linger, not places to heal. My oath is to heal the sick, not to prevent death." I felt this conversation solidified something between us: someday soon we would have to deal with the reality of David's future.

At a CDP meeting, everyone lamented their frustration. In a sense, each was saying, "I am helpless; it can't continue." I stated, "You are all where I was two years ago. David, you all, the family, and I cannot go on."

Although everyone nodded in agreement, no one wanted to come out and say what I had said or even admit it. Finally, Jackie said it: "My worst nightmare is seeing David sitting in the bubble and shaving."

When David returned Wednesday, October 17, he said, "I want to talk private—promise you won't tell. Why the press conference? Why am I on TV? Why am I special?"

"Because you live in an isolator."

"Well, I don't know why that should make me special—the bubble is my home."

"True, but people don't understand, so they're curious. You're not different, but living in a bubble is different."

"Yeah, I guess so. People don't know much about bubbles. I'm the expert on bubbles. I know more about bubbles than anyone else in the world."

"You can say that again."

He needed three words defined: "survive," "genetic," and "abortion"—the three words invariably spoken in any discussion of his case history.

"Survive means to remain alive—continue to live."

"Now that makes sense."

"Genetics has to do with genes and heredity. We inherit characteristics from our parents, like color of eyes."

"I got it."

"Abortion is when the embryo doesn't develop right and comes out of the mother before it grows into a baby."

"That's sad. What does that have to do with right to life and the anti-abortions signs?"

"There are two types of abortion. Spontaneous is one. The other is elective—a woman elects to have the embryo surgically removed."

"Why would she do that?"

"Lots of reasons—her health, a defective fetus, or she might not want a baby."

"It's too depressing. Let's discuss it some other time."

"Remember that neighbor kid who doesn't have a good brain? Well, he visited me and said, 'I had a nightmare last night. I was in the bubble with you.' I told him, 'Well, if you were in here with me, it truly would be a nightmare!' Can you imagine me having a retarded boy in here?"

The frequency and intensity of David's explosive rages increased. Afterwards, aghast, he was afraid people would leave and not come back. Several times he lashed out at Jackie, immediately caught himself, apologized, and pleaded, "Do you love me? Will you come back?"

Jackie visited with him late in the afternoon, and many a time she called me saying, "I'm afraid to leave him." I started going up to him after work. We ate dinner together, and he was content to entertain himself while I worked on my dissertation.

He said, "When I'm alone, each second is an hour. When you're here, each second is a second."

Jackie and I were at a total loss as to how to help him and our great fear was that he would burst out of the bubble in blind fury. She and I would have supported him in a rational decision to come out, but we couldn't have handled an impulse driven action instantly regretted.

We were disturbed over David's preoccupation with death, and fascination with fire. He drew giant flames to burn down the hospital or his home: After drawing the building on fire, he pretended to put it out by urinating on it.

David had Jackie and me drawing traffic signs again and again. In his own fantasy, signs seemed to be a symbolic way to work through his problems. Perhaps he relied on us to tell him how to stop and start. Possibly he used our sensors to clarify and objectively work through his anxieties and build in his own controls. Barry Molish had had some of the same thoughts to explain the absurd hide-and-go-seek game: "Every other person in the world has a place to hide, but he is always visible." He said David did not dare hide from anyone but me, because he knew I would never forget him.

Jackie and I understood the dynamics of David's angry behaviors, but we didn't know how to ease his pain. Deprived of investigating, trying out, changing, and controlling his world, he failed to achieve a sense of competence, independence, and self-worth. Feeling so powerless, he experienced constant fear, and the hostility built up. Any minor incident triggered the release of pent-up emotions in a torrent of displaced anger all out of proportion to the situation.

David paid a high price for security. Because of his absolute dependence, he dare not act on any angry feelings towards adults. His precarious situation never allowed him to anticipate the future or become a member of a group. A peer group for an eight-year-old is all-important—it allows him to reach out, touch lives, enjoy rewards, be appreciated, and have a goal to continue to grow.

Kids select their own friends, but David had no choice. He accepted whoever was brought to him. Any group activity he engaged in was contrived and artificial. To him, the future was bleak; he was a social outcast, isolated and alone. By necessity, he had to adopt a compliant, subservient, self-suppressing attitude, and this only intensified his antagonism and resentment.

Added to his sense of not belonging was the belief and reality that people were pulling away from him. He told me, "Everyone smiles too much, and I hate it when the nurses try to make me feel better." Potts found it difficult to hold back the tears when she looked at him. It was one thing to have a baby in a bubble, but to have a cognitively alert; sensitive, eight-year-old confined boy was different. He knew his growing up was hard on people and that the older he got, the more choices were denied him.

In an effort to divert David's attention, I started taking my son's paintings with me on my evening visits. The paintings fascinated him. He studied them for hours, commenting on every detail. The first one I took was called *Tranquility*. He chided, "You said Bill painted abstracts. This isn't abstract, it's real—a peaceful forest with trees and fluffy clouds." To another, a Maui landscape, he exclaimed, "Now that is not abstract, it is really real. It's *Hawaii Five-O!*"

Seeing Bill's most impressive painting he sighed, "Oh! Oh, my! That man is in agony. Why is he crying?"

"Bill painted *Agony* during a troubled time. It stays in the closet—it's too powerful and painful to look at. I've been told Bill captured a dying person's mottled skin to perfection."

Viewing the one I called *Happiness,* David commented, "Fish, balloons, flowers, clouds—everything pretty and happy, this one is sorta abstract."

In a strange, mystical way, my favorite painting made the greatest and most lasting impression on David. For him, it symbolized immortality. In this painting, which I call *Ethereal Beauty,* the palest imaginable lavenders and blues dominate. Firmly rooted columns extend from bottom to top. Airy delicate balls float among the columns and into clouds in a dark purple-blue sky.

Seeing this picture, David immediately cried out, "Eternity! That man is walking into eternity. It is beautiful. It's the most beautiful thing I ever saw." I had never noticed the shadowy figures walking into the yellow area.

I treasure my son's paintings, but somehow they held even more meaning for David. He was aware of every nuance Bill expressed and in that sense, they communicated.

It was ironic, because face to face, their conversations were stilted. David would ask lots of questions and then say, "Isn't it time for you to fly away from Houston?"

Bill told me: "I don't like talking with David—it's like being in a verbal duel, an adversarial situation in which I can never win. He speaks articulately and confidently on subjects I know he has limited or no knowledge about. He comes across as 'the expert'—once I lost an argument about my own car. I don't like feeling defeated by 'Little Brother' even though I am aware that, in part, my attitude springs from jealousy."

David's voice brought me back to the reality of his dying. "Mary, do you still keep *Eternity* hanging over your bed?"

I answered, "Yes," and thought to myself, and all I ever see is you, my love, entering into that sphere of eternity.

12.

THE THREE ALTERNATIVES

"Mary, I could never conceive what it would be like to be out of the isolator. Now, here I am, out. I'll tell you one thing, I didn't expect to be in a room like this doing nothing. Remember when I first thought about coming out?"

"Yes. It was about four years ago—you were eight."

"Yeah, I was afraid those psychiatrists would tell people I was crazy. Did they use the word crazy?"

"What did their report say?"

"No. The report was couched in psychoanalytic terms—the Oedipal stage, not prepared for latency and that stuff. Any psychiatrist or psychologist with knowledge of your case history could have written the same report without ever talking with you—anxious, and conflicts over being dependent."

"Remember what an awful time that was?" "How could I forget?"

In the winter and spring of 1980, the CDP meetings resembled a broken record—a litany of complaints about David's behavior, the family's passivity, and the inability to deal with the ever-increasing cracks in the bubbles.

It had been obvious to me for a long time that a new isolator system had to be designed. Several times I had proposed contacting Raymond Loewy, the industrial designer whose classic creations included the Coca-Cola bottle. He had described, as his most satisfying job, designing a comfortable living space for the astronauts. My suggestion was always vetoed—Loewy would want publicity and money. I argued that a man of his eminence, wealth, and age (over eighty) would do it for humane reasons. Gary Whitney knew Loewy, and he was certain he would donate his services, but the idea was never pursued.

A taller crib with two pairs of air inlets was ready in January. To prevent sagging, four giant rubber bands (the same kind used to secure the inside port caps) attached to the four corners of the crib were fastened to springs on ceiling hooks.

David stepped up his and my surveillance for cracks, which were hard to distinguish from creases. The ports' braces worked loose and the sleeves pulled out from under the tape. Finally, David declared, "It's a battle with the bubbles. They don't like me anymore and I haven't done anything to them." The carpenter shop reinforced the ports, solving the sleeve problems, but one mishap after another continued. At home he twice faced the ordeal of a three-hour power failure and had two big cuts out of big gloves; those ordered in February arrived in July. David, convinced the bubbles hated him and that everyone was tired of him, said, "One, two, three, four, I can't take any more."

David's psychological deterioration was now generally accepted. At the February 1980 CDP meeting the teachers described David's increased self-stimulating behaviors as interfering with his learning. Dr. Desmond surmised that David's anxieties had escalated and he had much difficulty maintaining self-quieting and self-control. Dr. Hansen suggested, "It is time to ask for help from a child psychiatrist in determining what is going on inside David's head—what is bothering him?"

For years, David had submitted to the ordeal of frequent blood drawings. The blood, aside from being used to monitor his physical condition, was studied by researchers far and near. Dr. Shearer's studies necessitated even more blood. In early years, when he was immobilized on a papoose board, blood drawing was easy. Now the procedure required his full cooperation.

During the October 1979 hospital stay, David's blood stopped during a routine drawing. He became upset, and after several attempts to stick him again, the nurses and he quit. He dreaded the next time and it turned into a disaster. They started at eight in the morning. At noon, David and the two nurses, totally spent, wringing wet with sweat and in tears, gave up.

"I'm humiliated to be seen like this," David said.

"He tried to control his hysteria and cooperate, but disintegrated. If he had just screamed and objected, I could have handled it," said Donna.

During the January stay, I gave advice, but resisted actually assisting blood drawing for several reasons: The early morning procedure interfered with my schedule at CDP; I didn't know what to do; and I'm squeamish at blood drawing, mine or anyone else's.

In March, the nurses refused to attempt to draw blood. I finally agreed to help. As usual, my presence calmed David but he piteously wailed, "It will hurt! She'll miss! My vein will stop!"—on and on.

"Donna, when you're all set, let him know," I ordered. "David, you count one, two, three, now. Then, Donna, do it." He hesitated counting twice, but in thirty minutes, the blood was drawn and there were no tears.

During the procedure, I recognized what was happening and realized that psychologist Albert Ellis's rational, cognitive approach was needed for success. That evening I explained, "David, you're awfulizing. You're saying, 'This blood drawing is awful, this is terrible, I can't stand it, it's awful, awful, awful.' You're not using your good mind, your cognition. You lose control because your awful feelings dominate what your good intelligence could take care of. The next time, you tell yourself, 'I don't like this. It might hurt a little, but I'm in control, and it will be over in a few minutes.' "

He immediately grasped the concept of awfulizing. The next week, the night before the blood drawing, he started to worry. I reminded, "The last time wasn't bad, and tomorrow you are going to be in complete control."

The next morning he hesitated for one moment. I touched his head with my gloved finger. "Remember, cognition."

He took a deep breath, thrust out his arm, and said "One, two, three, now!" He involuntarily shrieked when Donna adjusted the needle.

I said, "Remember we knew it would hurt a little bit." He calmed, and within five minutes the blood was in the tubes. Excited and proud of himself, he asked, "Was that a record time?" All agreed, and all of CRC applauded.

I said, "Such an excellent performance deserves a reward. What do you want?"

"A great big snail."

I bought two snails for his fish bowls, a mystery and a horned, and that evening he asked, "Did I do good?"

"You did. You were absolutely the bravest boy in the whole world. I don't know anyone who could have handled it better. Doesn't it feel great to have control?"

The next week, before his count, he interrupted, "Okay, Mary, that's enough of your calming words." From then on, I was present at the blood drawing. David did well, and it never took more than a few minutes. During the procedure, I stood between the supply and crib bubbles, with my arms in the gloves, carrying out my assignment peeling and holding the bandage.

David kept the crib and supply bubbles clean and orderly now. But he was a packrat. The playroom was his storage bin, and on the outside broken toys and papers were stacked everywhere. Nothing, not coercion, threats, or promises, moved him to discard one scrap of paper. For a boy whose whole environment was so tiny, this was a major problem. In desperation I sent a note to Dr. Shearer requesting he write an order—nothing new in unless something went out.

But the mess continued until a Sunday afternoon when my mother dropped by to see us. Junk was piled high on the windowsill, the TV, and the floor. Mother took one horrified look. "For heaven's sake, I can't come into this room, I'll break my neck. David, how do you walk in the playroom? I can't see the floor! Get busy and clean it up. Mary Ada, do something about the outside before I come back."

David snapped to attention. "Yes, ma'am."

David filled three pillowcases with trash from the playroom and allowed me to discard two large trash bags full of stuff from the outside. The broken tape recorder had to remain. When my mother returned, David stood with one hand on his hip grinning. Mother said, "This is better. I'll come in." With one forcefully issued, motherly command, she had accomplished what had stymied a team of professionals for years.

During David's March hospital stay, Carol Ann and Donna viewed the prototype of the redesigned space suit—the one scheduled to have been completed in January. David, furious with them for going to NASA, vehemently expressed opposition, "I'm angry because I had no part in this decision. I'm the one that has to get in it. Someone should have discussed it with me. I do have a legal right."

His parents ignored his protest—when the time came, he would get in and that was that. Plans were made for NASA to train the nurses to operate the new MBIS.

Despite the mounting tensions and problems, David and I had good times together in the spring of 1980. His interest in current events, social issues, the origins and future of mankind, and my dissertation made for engaging conversation. Once, as I struggled to write a paragraph, he said, "Stop. I'll help. Now, tell me exactly what you are trying to say." I did and he said, "That sounded fine. Write it down."

David continued to enjoy the fish, despite accidents. When one jumped out, he said, "He must be so afraid, being out of his home."

My son's letters, which David avidly read, described the customs of the two African tribes working for him, as well as his monkeys and his parrot. The natives believed Bill to be a magic juju man, because his chickens grew large and laid many eggs. The secret: he fed them, rather than making them scratch for their food as the Africans did. We mailed garden seeds to Bill, and he had great success with vegetables, but worms ate his melons. We phoned Texas A&M, and after David quizzed the agricultural scientist there, he ordered: "Telex Bill: Forget cantaloupes—they can't handle fruit flies." David became an expert on the African bush country from Bill's amazing escapades and tales.

David also began to take an interest in my finances. He learned about income tax from his father, a CPA. He volunteered, "My father can help you with your income tax." I turned over some of Bill's and my tax returns to David Sr. From then on, Little David took charge, and each year made certain I got everything ready in January.

David asked, "If you put all your money together would you have a hundred dollars?"

I replied, "More."

He asked, "A million?" I laughed. In time, he knew every detail of my investments.

The serious, provocative, side to our conversations involved David's striving to make some sense out of his world and somehow to cope better. He repeatedly said, "I don't understand what's going on or why."

However, he understood and clearly articulated his situation. "I'm different. I live in a bubble because of a genetic defect, SCID, inherited from my mother." He talked at length about decision making and repeatedly asked, "What decisions did you make today? How do you make a decision?"

"Decisions usually involve risks. You have to weigh each side—list in your mind the good and the bad, and then make a decision. You use judgment. Some people like making decisions, they quickly resolve the problem and come to a conclusion. Others go through life never making a decision, and then they live in misery, with constant frustration.

"Would you please tell me what was the biggest decision you ever made?"

"Leaving my marriage."

"Tell me, step by step, how you made that decision."

"The bad side was giving up security and the identity of 'Mrs.' and the institution of marriage. The good side was I could smile and do things I wanted to do."

After a long silence, David said, "Mary, you have been happy in your freedom. Haven't you?"

"Yes. I'll tell you what happened. I spent a lot of time awfulizing and feeling miserable, never truly understanding why. Every evening I walked Bunchy along the Bayou and often saw this young man. One day he said, 'If you looked up, you might see a star.' "

"Startled, I asked, "Is it that obvious?"

"I went into psychotherapy and was told, 'You like being miserable—if you didn't you would do something about it.' After I gained insight and realized the futility of trying to please and to be a perfect wife, I moved out. I became me, a me I like."

"Mary, turn around. Look. There's a star. Our star."

The last week in May, Carol Ann phoned, very disturbed at having learned Frank Weaver, of Baylor public relations, was leaving Baylor to move to Cincinnati. She had known him since before David was born, considered him a friend, and trusted his judgment. Now, after eight and a half years, Potts was the only one remaining from the original team.

When David came back to the hospital on June 4, everything came to a head. Nothing changed for the better. He looked troubled, worn, and sad. He said, "I didn't have enough air at home, and what I had was too hot. I wish they would set the thermometer low."

On the sixth, his parents and Dr. South visited him. After they left, he phoned and begged me to come. He hadn't eaten dinner and refused to eat for me, but talked. He said his mother was relieved that her sister had had a baby girl, not a boy—clearly, the sex-linked gene was an ongoing concern in Carol Ann's whole family. He talked about his great-grandmother having cancer. It was nearly midnight before he went to sleep.

Jackie and I were having almost identical nightmares of taking David out of the bubble and outside to play. Jackie said, "I'm trying to stuff him back through a port before someone discovers what I've done." In my dream, he and I were always running to get back before someone missed him. In those first two weeks in June when he was back at the hospital, Jackie and I didn't have one moment's peace. The long evening hours with him drained me. It seemed as though he survived on my energy alone.

I decided that the day David next went home, June 18, I would compose a letter explaining my fear that he would burst out in a rage, as well as explaining our frustration and helplessness in the face of David's pain. In essence, I wanted to say that David, Jackie, Donna, and I had reached the limit. But first, I wanted to discuss it with Dr. Feigin.

Before I had a chance to say anything, Dr. Feigin beat me to it. "There is no cure for David—he cannot continue, the whole situation is intolerable for everyone," he told me.

He and Dr. Shearer were to meet with public relations and administration from both Baylor and the hospital to lay out the alternatives that were to be presented to the parents. He felt public relations would strongly object to any change in David's status, and he wanted my support and help in answering their questions.

It was one thing to discuss my feelings, David's future, and what had to be done with Dr. Feigin, Jackie, or Dr. Shearer, but to make a public formal statement!

The meeting was held on June 17, 1980. As I entered, Dr. Feigin took my arm and seated me next to him. Others in the group included Ralph Frede (head of Baylor public relations) and his assistant, Kaylen Fry. The hospital representatives were Pat Kiley (public relations), Ruth Sylvester, R.N. (administration), Dr. Desmond, and three CRC nurses, Donna, Betty, and Shannon.

Dr. Shearer was to meet with the parents at nine the following day, and for the first time lay out the reality of it all.

David's situation and three alternatives:

David could continue in the present isolator for probably another two or three years.

He could receive some type of transplant to reconstitute his deficient immune system—a fetal thymus, fetal liver, or an incompatible bone marrow.

He could be a removed from the isolator and given immunoglobulin replacement therapy and conventional antibiotic to resist infection. Dr. Shearer would recommend this alternative to the parents.

He further explained that the reason for the decision being made now was that the people working with David, the psychiatric evaluation, and the psychiatrist working with Carol Ann indicated a deterioration in the boy's mental status was obvious but denied problems in the family. He said, "Mary had planned to dictate a letter tomorrow, after David went home, about her feelings that we had possibly reached the limit."

He continued, "One big problem is the family's loyalty and trust in the original doctors. We have no control over what these three might do."

To a question on life expectancy, Dr. Feigin explained that, at best with a transplant David would have two years and, probably, with the antibiotic therapy about nine months. He and Dr. Shearer again both emphasized that they couldn't say this, in fact, because there was no precedent. They had no actual knowledge and were basing their estimates on statistics of other transplants. Again, Dr. Feigin said, "No decision is being made, and no action is being taken yet."

Money for maintenance was discussed. Dr. Feigin said there was always the issue of money—realistically, when the government made a site visit we could not justify keeping David in his environment on a research basis. However, he wanted it made clear that no decision about David's future would ever be made on the basis of money alone.

Though it was swept under the rug at this meeting, the issue of money would loom large from this point on. Increasingly, researchers were pointing out that the research value of this "project" had been exhausted.

Mr. Frede inquired, "How will David be told? How will you get him out of the bubble?"

Dr. Shearer answered, "That is a whole other problem and not what we are dealing with today."

I interjected, "We can deal with that, but I agree with Dr. Shearer, it shouldn't be considered at this point." I was already on complete overload. This topic would have crumpled me.

I recalled having talked with the physicians about this before, and someone having said, "He will come out for Mary." I wanted to bolt the meeting, run away, and never come back. Didn't anyone realize what this was doing to me?

I must have looked as ghastly as I felt because Dr. Feigin repeatedly whispered, "Mary, are you all right? Are you sure?"

"My God," I was thinking. "How could I ever ask my love to come out to die? He's a part of me. He can't die. I won't let him die."

Then I heard my own mother's words to a friend: "You have it wrong. Mary Ada doesn't worry about David's dying, she worries about David's living."

My anguish increased when my thoughts went beyond my own grief and ambivalence to the next day. How would Carol Ann and David Sr. take this shattering blow to their hope and faith? I would have given anything to be naive about parental reaction, but from my work with parents of handicapped children, I knew the impact of Dr. Shearer's honesty would be devastating. I relived experiences of telling parents what they did not want to hear. I recalled every grief reaction imaginable: tears, complete denial, anger, and shock. Then, somehow, all the hundreds of faces I had witnessed faded away, and I remembered only one mother and how she lashed out at me: "I knew you were going to say my son was retarded, but when you said it out loud, you took away my last hope, and I hate you for that."

The affection between Carol Ann and me had grown. By this time, the strong bond between us included more than our mutual love for a child. The Carol Ann I knew was not a beautiful facade, but a stoic woman of integrity who coped with what I viewed as an impossible situation. Admittedly, I was often annoyed by her procrastination, passivity, tardiness, and refusal to look beyond the surface. But then I would think, "What if I were in her position, how would I handle it?" I probably couldn't have. She was surviving and doing it with dignity and grace.

After all, it was Carol Ann who had drawn me into the case six years before when she had perceived the special relationship between her son and me and mentioned it to Dr. Montgomery. She believed that God had sent me to her and David. She often told me that each morning she prayed and thanked God that I loved her son.

The first poignant moment between us had been when she was teary and upset at David's crying when returning to the hospital. I had said, "That's the way it should be. A three-year-old should cry when he's going to be away from his mother for a long time. He'll be all right."

Relieved somewhat of her guilt, she had thanked me for giving her freedom and started making short out-of-town visits. I had said, "I give you permission to go and to enjoy—and not feel guilty."

She had laughed and said, "No one ever told me anything like that before."

Our usual greeting to each other on David's arrival or departure from the hospital was, "Here he is—he is all yours." I was exhausted by the time David returned home, and Carol Ann was just as exhausted when he was ready to come back to the hospital. She once said that she did fine until that last two days. I could empathize with that because usually the last few days he was at the hospital I wondered if I could make it until he was gone. We both knew that our being able to say this to each other did not diminish our love for him or our affection for each other.

Now, walking away from the meeting, all these memories and thoughts bombarded me—there was absolutely no escape. I had to finish the workday and then face the evening with David. Was there any way to take it all back, any way to stop tomorrow?

That night I didn't close my eyes, let alone sleep, but the next morning I seemed to have energy. The blood drawing went quickly and easily. Fortunately for me, Katherine had come along with her parents, so David was busy talking with her, as their parents met with Dr. Shearer and Dr. Desmond.

When Carol Ann came from the meeting she said hello to David and me, then tears welled in her eyes. I took her to the nurses' lounge and she asked, "You know why Dr. Shearer wanted to meet with us?"

"Yes—"

"I always knew in the back of my mind that this day would come, but I expected David to decide, not me or my husband. If he asked to come out of the isolator, we would not stand in his way."

David Sr. came in and held her.

"I'll tell David you have a headache," I said. "I really don't feel well at all," she replied.

Fortunately, only Potts had witnessed Carol Ann's outburst. Carol Ann had once told me that she couldn't bear the thought of anyone seeing her cry.

I went back to David and said, "I know you expected your mother to ride in the van with you, but you have three here today to choose from: Why don't you decide who rides with you?" I knew that he would pick Katherine. The rest of the workday was a blur for me. When I got home I crawled in bed to cry and mercifully fell quickly asleep.

13.

ST. JUDE

I've awakened. It's dark. This isn't my bed. I'm dreaming. "Mary—you dozed off."

David is in a bed beside mine; he's out of the bubble. His parents made the decision. Muddled, I thought, "That's a young man talking, not a little boy." Fully awake, I realized it was February 1984, but my thoughts drifted back to the evening of June 18, 1980, when I awoke and phoned Carol Ann.

"I can't stop crying," Carol Ann told me. "I appreciated Dr. Shearer's honesty—no one has ever been honest with me before. I can't stand to be in the room with David yet, but it's all working out okay; some friends are here and Big David is cooking dinner."

"I couldn't cry at work, but I've made up for it since I've been home," I said.

"I'm not going to try to make a decision until I stop crying. I'll need some help. I would like to talk to Dr. Shearer more, but that would be imposing."

"You're wrong; feel free to call him any time—at home or the office. We are all hurting. Dr. Feigin and Dr. Shearer have agonized over this and explored every possibility."

"Before I make a decision, I want to talk to Dr. Wilson and Dr. Montgomery."

"You can't make a decision without talking with your husband."

"His only comment was, 'No quack psychiatrist is going to tell me what to do with my son!' This afternoon I found some peace sitting in church and praying, but the priest came in. He's never been helpful; he's too compassionate. Whenever I discuss Little David with him, he cries and I have to comfort him."

"Call me or Dr. Shearer."

"I will. I promise. Before David was born, the obstetrician advised a glass of wine. I'll have one if I can't sleep. Please call me tomorrow. I hate to call when you're busy."

The next morning I suggested to Dr. Shearer that he call Carol Ann. "She really wants to reach out to you, but doesn't feel free to do so."

That evening, Carol Ann called. "I thought that somehow if I could just go to sleep that I'd wake up in the morning and things would be better—but they weren't."

"It's like a bad dream," I said. "I keep thinking I'll wake up and it won't be true."

"That's it exactly. Big David didn't sleep either. I know he'd been crying because his eyes were so red. We look at the hurt in each other's eyes and try to protect each other. I don't know whether we can ever talk. I'm grateful for Dr. Shearer's call. I'm to talk with him on Wednesday."

"You should talk with your husband."

"I always thought David would ask to come out," Carol Ann said quietly. "You'd be proud of me. I've put myself together, at least on the surface. I wish you could see me."

"Would you like me to drive out?"

"I'd really like that, but how would we explain it to David? Could you come on the weekend?"

"I'll come Sunday afternoon."

"I feel so numb. Is this the way I'm supposed to feel?"

"In grief we go through stages—shock or numbness, denial, and anger."

"Anger?"

"Yes, everyone gets angry in a time of loss or grief. I see it in the parents I work with. They direct their anger at each other, or me, or the physician."

"You know, it's funny that you said that. When my baby died, Dr. Klish was taking care of him, and I thought he was the ugliest man in the world. I never understood those feelings. I guess that's what it was. When Dr. Klish came out to the house for David when he swallowed the coin and was so kind working with him, I decided he wasn't really ugly."

After we had discussed grief reactions and anger at length, I finally said, "You should expect one of your next reactions to be anger. Just don't direct it at me."

"I would never do that. I've always been grateful to you; you've given me the freedom to do things because you take care of my little boy when he's at the hospital.

"What do I tell Katherine? She knows something is wrong."

"You know her better than I—follow your mother's instinct. You'll know when it's the right time. Just remember, she is probably conjuring up things in her mind that are worse than the truth."

"You're right. She asked if my husband and I were getting a divorce."

Carol Ann and I talked nearly every day. She and her husband did not discuss the three alternatives and it drove me crazy.

On Sunday, the family greeted me with open arms and kisses. Every time David Sr. and I started to talk, friends dropped in. Carol Ann was tired and torn between David's needs and those of Katherine and her husband. Eventually, we had a chance to speak in private.

"If my son stays in, I don't know how much longer I can make it, but taking him out means killing him," Carol Ann said. "If given even the smallest hope, I wouldn't hesitate to say 'out'. I don't want to be unrealistic, but at the same time, I cannot make it without hope, even if it's small."

"I remember Raphael Wilson saying, "Hope is what maintains everyone!" I didn't voice my belief that hope can be agony—struggling against reality and the inevitable can destroy a person. The thought of David staying in is excruciating, but the thought of his dying is unbearable."

David, delighted to see me, didn't question my visit. He told me, "I'm pondering over making a decision." Naturally, no one had told him about the three choices, but David was extraordinarily intuitive, and had figured out that the people around him were discussing the possibility of taking him out of the bubble.

It would have been so easy to suggest, "Just say, 'I want to come out.'" But I could not do it.

Carol Ann phoned on Tuesday to make certain I would be free to meet with her after she talked with Dr. Shearer, and she began reflecting on the past. "Before David II was conceived, my husband and I discussed the risks involved and decided to chance it. We weren't trying to replace the baby. I don't know if you understand this—it wasn't just to fill the loss. When we married, we planned to have at least three children, and we wanted to continue. That was the last time we discussed anything—including putting the baby in the isolator."

Carol Ann disclosed her plan of action. "After I talk with Dr. Shearer tomorrow, I'm going to phone Dr. Montgomery, then Drs. Wilson and Bealmear, and last, if at all, Dr. South—her reaction is the only one I can predict. She'll be emotional—I don't know whether I'm up to that. I dread talking with Dr. Wilson because I cannot resist him; he can persuade me to do anything. He did before, and he can now. My mother and he are the two people who can do this to me."

"Listen, I understand," I said. "But this decision must be made by you and your husband."

The next day, Carol Ann called me from Dr. Shearer's office, and we met in Dr. Feigin's office for privacy. "My mother just called; my grandmother is dying. I must go to San Antonio immediately. I appreciate Dr. Shearer's honesty, and I don't want you to think I'm not being rational with all these tears, but I am going to follow his advice. To continue with my son in the bubble is not fair to Katherine or my husband, and I can't see David being subjected to those painful procedures."

For the first time, I voiced my opinion. "This is best. I don't know how much longer any of us, including your son, will have the energy to continue."

"Dr. Shearer offered some small hope. He doesn't know exactly what will happen if David comes out."

"Talk with your husband!" I pleaded.

"What should I tell David about his great-grandmother?" "The truth."

That evening Carol Ann phoned to tell me that her grandmother had died. She wanted me to spend the weekend with Little David. Donna and her husband were staying at the house.

On Friday when I arrived, David talked at length about his mother's and his own sadness. Then he asked question after question about funerals and wills.

Carol Ann called on Monday to thank me. She was exhausted. "David's adult attitude toward my grandmother's death is amazing. His understanding of my feelings and words of comfort eased my grief. I'm very proud of my son."

The following Tuesday, when Carol Ann called to talk about David's upcoming return to the hospital, I was working with a child. The next day I called to apologize for "hanging up on her," but David Sr. answered. He was hostile.

"Before making any decisions about my son's future, I want to talk to lots of people and have things in writing! Little David, himself, has to have a part in the decision," he said.

"I concur, especially with the latter," I said.

Thursday morning, July 17, Carol Ann came to my office to inquire about her son's first evening back. She confided, "I am so sorry that Dr. South is coming tonight. I'm not ready to talk, but she just called again to tell me she is bringing a technician. I take this as a sign from God not to discuss Little David. I want to stick to my plan. She will be on the end of the list, if at all."

Late in the afternoon I spent time with David; he was in a good mood.

That evening the nurse greeted me with, "He's in a terrible mood."

"You're supposed to be my friend. Where were you when she was here? How dare you leave me alone with her and that man? I am very angry at you."

"I didn't know you needed me. All I can say is I'm sorry. I am pleased that you were able appropriately to confront me with your anger."

As we fixed a new fishbowl, David asked, "What is Dr. Shearer planning for me? Do you know?"

"Well, I know he has said there is no miracle pill, as everyone had hoped, and also he realizes that you cannot stay in the bubble forever, so he is working on something in between."

"Oh, that seems logical."

When I related this conversation to his mother, she said, "All I can say is I'm glad he asked you, not me. I couldn't have handled it."

The next weekend, Carol Ann told me that she and her husband had finally talked. She was pleased that the hospital stay had been extended a week.

Sunday, August 3, David phoned. "I'm frantic: my parents still don't answer the phone. Last night you said they probably went to a party. They're still not at home. I've called everybody. They've left—they're gone forever."

I was puzzled. Carol Ann always told me when they would be away. The only explanation was they had gone out of town to meet with the three original doctors.

The next two weeks were hell. Carol Ann didn't call, and I didn't feel free to call her. One day at noon, Dr. Feigin caught up with me in the hall and asked where I was going.

"Out for a walk. I've got to get out of the building. This is taking over my life."

"This is all very difficult for you, I know. If you want out, I understand. It will be all right, but I want you to stay in this with us. There is a limit to what you or anyone can take. It's all-consuming and leaves room for nothing else."

On August 20, David's parents told Dr. Shearer that they had met with Drs. Montgomery, South, and Wilson and that they had decided to keep David in the isolator until some new therapy was discovered that would offer a cure without risks and suffering.

The decision did not surprise me; I had known that David Sr. would make this choice. In their traditional patriarchal family, the loss of a son was the ultimate catastrophe. David Sr. once told me that since he had no brother his son absolutely had to carry on the family name. David's death would be more than the loss of a loved child; it would be the end of the family.

Donna took vacation from August 14 through 25 and hoped to recover from all the trauma. When she returned, she phoned and asked to meet.

"I can't take it any more—not being able to help David and the parents' hostility. I want you to know that if David had come out I would have stayed until the end; nothing could have made me leave him. But I intend to resign at the end of the year."

We talked at length. I understood her distress and said, "I envy you—it's too late for me. I can't leave him."

David returned to the hospital on Monday, September 8. He phoned at half past five. "Be here at seven. I have several problems to talk over."

My apprehension about the talk proved to be unfounded. He merely wanted to clear things through me—his way of checking or testing reality.

"I know of the developments—Dr. Shearer doesn't have a cure. Mary, I know what your decision would be."

"The decision was for your parents, not me, to make."

"Well, I'll tell you one thing, I'll have to be the one to make the decision."

I took a vacation day on Friday and holed up in my office to write. A distraught Donna phoned. "Come up right now—we need help before the photographers get here. David is shattered and can't stop crying. His father says he must wear the St. Jude medal his grandparents bought."

I stopped by Dr. Feigin's office. "Donna called for help—it's a fiasco up there. Do we have to have the photos?"

He stated emphatically, "Yes, with all the pressures the least we can get by with are stills. Go on up and get them."

Hazel Haby of public relations, in a tizzy, approached, "You have to." "Look, I talked with Dr. Feigin—you'll get your pictures." Donna and I conversed briefly.

"Can't we talk with his father?" I asked.

"That's the problem—he did, and now he has no choice, he has to wear it."

"Is the medal the special birthday present to be opened right before the photo session—the anticipated gold wristwatch?"

"Yes, was he ever disappointed."

David was, indeed, in a state. "I can't go on. I can't have my pictures made. Everything is terrible: I have no choices, no way out." He frantically demanded, "In the gloves!" I held him, and finally the sobs subsided.

"I can't have my picture in the newspaper wearing jewelry.... People will think I'm crazy," he moaned. "I hate jewelry. What am I going to do? My dad said I must wear it. Not only will people think I'm crazy—don't you think I don't know about the Saint of the Hopeless? I watch the Memphis marathon on TV, and I know all about St. Jude. Anyway, boys don't wear jewelry."

"Settle down, we'll think of something." "No. No. No way—there's no choice."

"With the gold and silver design on your yellow shirt no one will notice the medal," I suggested.

"They will. I can't disappoint my parents and my grandparents, and I can't have my picture in the paper wearing jewelry!"

"Stop crying—"

Donna knocked on the door and motioned me out. Hazel Haby had learned the reason for David's storm. Flustered and agitated she grabbed my shoulder, "Do you realize the implications of our releasing pictures with him wearing a St. Jude medal? I can see the *National Enquirer* headlines—"Bubble Boy Wears the Medal of the Hopeless." Do you understand what I am saying?"

"Goddammit, yes!" I shouted. I went back in David's room, slamming the door closed.

"What did they want? Are the photographers here?" he asked.

"No. They wanted to make sure you'd be ready when they were. Listen to me. No more tears. We're going to work this out. What exactly did your father say?"

"He said I had to wear it."

"Did he say where?"

"No."

"Well...?"

"Oh! I knew you would come up with the solution. You always do. Help me hook it." We hooked the chain and tucked the medal under his shirt. "Maybe I'll pull the chain out from under the shirt so they can see it a little bit, but no one will know it's jewelry."

"David, we've got to do something about your eyes. Drink some water. Wet a washcloth to wipe your eyes."

He lay down for a few minutes with a wet cloth across his eyes and then combed his hair. The photographers knocked on the door and asked to come in. David unconditionally stated, "Okay, but only if she stays."

One photographer immediately noticed the little bit of chain showing and asked, "What is that? Bring it out—let's see."

I held both hands up in one photographer's face and screamed, "Drop it!" The photographer, fortunately, did not persist.

David refused to smile but finally struck a bargain. "If you take a picture of Mary, one where she looks terrible, just awful, and then give the picture to me and nobody else, I'll smile." The Venetian blind broke when they pulled it up for more light, so during the session I stood on the windowsill holding the blind up, and that's where I was when they took my picture. After all of the horrendous prelude, the photos of David actually turned out beautifully, especially those of him feeding his fish.

Later, Carol Ann told Donna that if she had been there David would have worn the necklace—there would have been no problem because "it is a child's duty to please his parents." Very soon after the photo session, the necklace disappeared. Years later, it reappeared in the hem of the playroom curtain.

On September 16, Drs. Shearer, Desmond, and Hansen discussed the psychiatric report and the correspondence from the leading immunologists with the parents. Carol Ann told me Dr. Hansen had answered no to her husband's questions: "Is David psychotic?" and "Can he get better without treatment?" She was angry with Dr. Hansen for evading her one important question: "Is the isolator the cause of the basic problem?"

David planned a "private" ninth birthday party for best friends at noon on Thursday, September 18, 1980. He wrote six invitations and with Potts's help selected the refreshments. On Tuesday, he became perturbed when he learned his mother had invited others, but on Wednesday his spirits lifted.

Thursday, I was extra busy and I could not get up to CRC at noon. Donna and others left messages: "David is crying and refusing to let us cut the cake until you get here."

Carol Ann called for me and then called Dr. Desmond, "Tell Mary to stop working and come to the party."

Dr. Desmond, already incensed by Carol Ann's behavior since June, came into my office furious. "She can't go around giving me orders and demanding your time! I am going to the party in your place."

I phoned David. "I can't get away. I will be there at five, and we'll celebrate then."

"I'll make sure they save enough of everything, and I'll keep your cake and ice cream right here."

At five, when I walked in, he burst into tears, "But, Mary, didn't you know that the only reason I planned the party was so you could share my birthday with me? Dr. Desmond and that woman came."

"What woman?"

"You know. That woman that works for 'she'."

We both cried, and after being in my arms for a while, he requested I eat my cake and my melted ice cream. All the other food was gone.

The next day he cried when he left to go home and said, "I love you—please call on my birthday."

Donna introduced Lynn Franklin, R.N., her replacement, at the October 14 CDP meeting. While we waited for Arden Richardson and Dr. Coburn, the school psychologist, to arrive, Donna summarized David's violent opposition to the space suit.

Donna: He emphatically states he will not get in the suit. I tried to talk to Carol Ann about his protest. She said, "I do not want to discuss it—when the time comes my son is going to get into the suit no matter what." She feels it will be an embarrassing situation for her if he doesn't get in it. The family doesn't realize the problems we have, like the episode with the St. Jude medal.

Dr. Shearer: The parents think the suit is of great value. However, the value is not worth the hospital personnel effort and time. Currently, it may be ready in January. Mary, how long has it taken him to get into the suit before? Mary: The fastest was fifty minutes. I am out of the space suit deal. I will have no part in it. Before David went home, he extracted a promise from me not to coerce him. He said, "I know what you are going to say—I might change my mind so we should leave the door open. I have absolutely no intention of changing my mind. You must promise because I know if you decide I have to get in the suit I will." I promised, but I also told him if he changed his mind I would help him.

Donna expressed her, Jackie's, and my concerns that David was not looking forward to his favorite holiday, Halloween. Jackie suggested,

"Perhaps the costume his mother is planning is like the space suit—after all the preparations and anticipation, where does he go?"

When Arden and Dr. Coburn arrived, Dr. Shearer said, "The purpose of the meeting is to discuss the psychiatric evaluation. The report has been given to the parents, and the parents' explicit permission was elicited to share the report with Mrs. Richardson and the team. I am placing the burden on you that the meeting be entirely confidential." He reminded us of the press releases by the psychoanalyst and further stated, "The purpose is that we have grave concerns and feel that people like you who are working with David need to be informed, with the idea of helping him under very adverse environmental conditions."

Dr. Hansen stated, "David is in an isolated state and there is deviant behavior. I attempted to get a cross-sectional view from new people and not use people like Mary who is so involved with the child." He described the evaluators. An outside psychiatrist, who knew nothing of the history, consulted twice for a total time of five hours and gave a fresh look at the situation. The results were, "David was not psychotic, but his psychological development had been arrested, and he was not in the full latency stage."

Jackie and I looked at each other, dumbfounded. This is the psychiatric evaluation? This is introductory psychology!

Hansen: Treatment is urgent. At the present time, David has not mastered the skills required for the latency period, so, therefore, he doesn't have the skills to enter the puberty stage and to oppose his parents.

Desmond: David is showing marked changes in facial structure and musculature. He may be entering adolescence. (Dr. Hansen appeared startled.)

Donna: This last week, David has expressed an interest in female anatomy; he wants cutouts of nude girls from "girly" magazines. He also stated there were advantages to having a girl nurse and remarked about a new nurse's "interesting legs".

Desmond: Where is he getting all this from?

Mary: It was quite evident last spring but then subsided. He sees it on cable TV and the "soaps." Also, he knows the shock value of his risqué comments.

Arden: The family situation is unusual. I don't mean to be derogatory, but to me, Carol Ann has developed a role as the "bubble baby mother." She is dressed like she stepped out of a fashion magazine any time you go to the house. Her role is completely surrounded by this Boy in the Bubble and the father doesn't seem to fit into the scene—he's on the periphery. I worry about Katherine and feel things are not as secure and stable as they appear.

Mary: Let's face it. He's not a cute baby bouncing around in a bubble. He's quite awkward.

Jackie: I'm really concerned about this adolescence, and I don't know how to help him.

Hansen: David's in the dependent-versus-independent-from-mother stage.

Mary: He is aware of being totally dependent on people for his existence, but he feels ambivalent toward his mother. He loves her but knows exactly why he's in the bubble.

Jackie: Yes, I've been aware of his feelings toward his mother for some time. As for my own feelings, I'm confused as to how to help him. It's been four years now, and I can't give him any assistance. He's at the puberty stage on one hand, and yet there he is, a child with a potty chair. It's so much like the parallel of raising a retarded child. He has all the problems that any adolescent has, but he doesn't have any of the tools to deal with them—just like a retarded child doesn't have the cognitive ability to deal with the problems.

Hansen: He exerts considerable pressure on the pubic area. Just when did this start?

Jackie: Six or eight months ago, wasn't it Mary?

Mary: Yes. The problem is he gets so upset and he has no calming mechanism.

Hansen: Yes, he's going into adolescence without having adequate latency skills.

Jackie: I have dealt with children who were going to die the next day, and I've felt adequate. I could do something with them. With David, I feel totally inadequate. I just don't know how to handle it. I don't know what to do.

Donna: Dr. Hansen, maybe you could give us some practical advice on how to deal with these matters.

Coburn (after no comment from Hansen):
People are at a handicap when they deal with him. We look at everything through our perspective, and David's perspective is certainly from a completely different viewpoint. (Dr. Hansen left.)

Jackie: It's just, almost a sheer management problem. He's at the toddler stage in so many things. It's like he says, "Catch me if you can" or "Try to make me."

Mary: I agree.

Arden: The school people tell me he behaves quite well. I'll tell you what I did when we had so much trouble. I went to the house, and Carol Ann left. David zipped into the playroom saying, "I won't. You can't make me." When I asked him where he ate and went to the bathroom he said, "Why ask dumb questions? You know." I told him that I was going to sit and wait until he crawled through the connection to eat or urinate, and then I was going to hit him over the head with a stick. He laughed and said I wouldn't dare do that and break the bubble. He was shocked when I said I didn't care, my only job was to educate. He came up to work. I don't think he ever told his mother.

Jackie: I don't like the way they use guilt to manage him.

Mary: They simply do not understand. They believe children are supposed to please their parents.

Jackie: Well, school is the only normal thing. Arden: Medically, Dr. Shearer, is there any change?

Shearer: No treatment is available that is acceptable to the parents. Previous doctors who have maintained a close relationship are still considered David's doctors by the parents. Although these doctors are no longer engaged in David's care, the parents listen to them and believe they know what is best. These physicians insist that maintaining him in his present isolation is the correct thing to do.

Arden: Several years ago, Carol Ann told me they had no control because of the high cost of keeping David. Who does pay?

Shearer:	The government grant to CRC pays for most of it. The hospital and the Ladies Auxiliary have added to the fund. We are actually at the point where funds may be stopped.
Arden:	What will you do if the funds are stopped? Shearer: The parents are aware of this possibility and have indicated that they will make an appeal to the public. A friend, who is a good friend of the President's, has assured them that they can get money from private foundations.
Arden:	Why can't he stay at the home all of the time? Does he have to come back to the hospital?
Shearer:	Yes, it is necessary for some blood work. Donna: The parents are really moving away from him.
	I feel they're almost rejecting him. It used to be when he came back to the hospital it would be a big to-do. Carol Ann would stay two hours. Now she doesn't even wait for him to be hooked up. It's come in, goodbye, and gone. Also, they're not visiting and just not doing anything.
Coburn:	Is he feeling as if he's being rejected?
Mary and Jackie:	Yes.
Donna:	Yes, he's very aware of it.
Arden:	Well, if you'll remember, some time ago I thought he should stay home more. Maybe it could be four weeks at home and one week at the hospital.
Mary:	How about six and two? Arden: That sounds good.
Mary:	Arden, did I hear you correctly? You are officially recommending six weeks at home and two weeks at the hospital?
Arden:	Yes, certainly I'm recommending six weeks at home and two weeks at the hospital.
Desmond:	I think the meeting is over.

Dr. Shearer thanked Arden and Dr. Coburn for attending and said that it was nice to have met them. After the meeting, Arden and Dr. Coburn talked to me. She felt there were real problems at home and wanted my opinion. I told her, "I think you know more about what is going on than I.

David Sr. has expressed anger toward me, and I haven't had any contact with them for two months."

Dr. Coburn said, "I have no intention of becoming involved in the case, but if you need help or want assistance, feel free to call me. I'll be glad to help you." This made me feel good.

I ate lunch with David on the day he returned, October 16. He seemed happy to be back and showed me Princess Leia, a beautifully dressed and coiffured doll based on the *Star Wars* character.

That evening, I walked into a violent, passionate tantrum. Leia's hair was messed up; he tried to re-comb it but couldn't. I did no better with the tiny doll combs through the gloves. Eventually, together, we managed to get her hair fixed to his satisfaction and moved on to hide-and-go-seek.

Later I read the note on the nurse's chart: "David's so upset about a doll it took Mary forty-five minutes to calm him." The next few days he continued to be in an irascible mood. He refused to eat and didn't even want food put in the supply. A few evenings later, David was able to speak rationally:

"God, how did I get in this fix, and how do I get out of it? Why am I afraid of so many things? Why am I afraid of her (Leia) when she is so little? I can hold her in one hand yet I'm so afraid of her. I'm going crazy. It's the only answer. I must be crazy. Why else would I be afraid of her and blame her for everything?"

"You are not crazy. Understanding feelings or the mind is complicated. It's terrible to live with anger. When we are always frustrated, hostility builds up and we have to get rid of it in a safe way—a way that allows us to maintain our self-respect. Any threat to our self-worth or adequacy is a threat to our very existence, and we have to protect ourselves. This is getting too deep."

"No. No. I'm getting it—go on."

An explanation of psychological defenses ensued. I said that people deal with problems or emotions in two basic ways—directly, by using their cognitive ability, or with unconscious devices called ego defense mechanisms. For example: Denial—we escape from or evade a painful truth by denying it exists. Projection—we blame others for our difficulties or attribute to others our own unacceptable thoughts or wishes. Displacement—we shift our anger from the person we are mad at to another or an object. Everyone employs all of these defenses at one time or another. Under severe stress, we tend to exaggerate the ones we normally use, and that's when we get in trouble.

"Let me go over those types and meanings," David said. He proceeded to give a remarkably accurate recap of what I had just explained. "How does being crazy fit into all this?"

"If we never attempt to solve a problem and exclusively use one or two defenses to cope, we get into delusions and never know if a threat is real or imagined. We are removed from reality or the real world."

"You started off with denial, projection, and displacement because you think that's what I use the most. Right? What are your main defenses? They're not the same as my three. I've never heard you accuse or blame anybody."

"I'm not sure," I said. "Probably repression and fantasy. That's enough psychology, I want to discuss something else—I intend for the next few months to be peaceful because I'm going to graduate. No more postponing my dissertation. It wears me out to calm you down and to worry about you."

"Yeah, me too."

"I have plans. Bill wants bids on rice for Mohammed Faruku, an entrepreneur he is working with in Nigeria. I don't know anything about rice. I talked to the people at The Rice Council. You're going to have to help me with this rice—bidding stuff. You already know a lot about the stock market. I'm going to subscribe to *The Wall Street Journal*, then you can keep up with my stock portfolio. I want our time together to be fun and productive, and that's the way it's going to be from now on."

"Sounds okay to me, but don't think I don't know what you're doing. You think you can keep me from going crazy. Let's face it—the time might come when...."

"Stop it. You are not going to go crazy. I refuse to give you permission to go crazy."

In October, depleted and exhausted, I went to Hillsboro, Missouri, to visit my cousin Anita and to rest. In a return to my childhood, I walked in the woods, looked at the beautiful leaves, and picked "farewell summers" — exquisite, but silly lavender flowers that didn't know they were supposed to bloom in the spring. I gained strength and the determination to go on.

14.

THE THREE DOCTORS RETURN

"Mary, we haven't done anything with your investments since before Christmas. You know when this is all over, you're going to have to handle them by yourself."

I thought, why don't you use the word die? Why don't I?

David went on, "One good thing, Bill's not in Africa trying for rice deals. My father is the only one who believed we bid on all that rice."

"That was long ago. You were so angry about Donna's plans to leave and the new schedule."

On November 5, 1980, Donna went to David's home to put in supplies and reported, "I never saw him so angry. He could barely contain his emotions enough to talk. He pounded his fists, held his breath, and screamed, 'I don't like the idea; six weeks at home is too long! I get bored! Frankly, it's more exciting at the hospital. You must remember, I have lots of friends there. I need change. If you want to keep me happy, make it five at home and three at the hospital. I've disappointed Mom by not liking the schedule. Even though I'm very sorry about that, I don't want the new schedule. If I go along with it to please her, I will disappoint myself.'"

At Dr. Feigin's request, I attended the November 19 meeting with the three original doctors. Larry Taber, M.D., was invited because he knew Dr. South well and his presence might ease the tension. Also, the president of Baylor was sending a representative. Dr. Feigin sat at the head of the table with Drs. Shearer and Montgomery on his right and Drs. Desmond, South, and Wilson on his left. I walked past Raphael; he took my hand and leaned forward for his customary kiss on my cheek. Despite this friendly gesture, the room was already full of bitter tension. Dr. Wilson disputed the "superficial examination." He had seen David and felt the boy's deterioration was being overstated.

"Raphael, you haven't spent more than a few minutes with David in the last three years—your visits are a hello and goodbye!" I snapped. While I described David's pain, despair, and feelings of hopelessness, Dr. Wilson stared at the corner of the ceiling.

Finally, he rebuked me: "You are overstating the case and really don't have David's best interest at heart."

Livid, I retaliated: "Raphael, you of all people should never question my affection for this child!"

He backed down. "The parents have told me how important you are to David and to them, but I don't believe things are as bad as you say."

Furious, I did not care who was in the room or what I said. "I know David. You don't."

As I started to bolt out of my chair in anger, Larry Tabor interjected, "I'm no psychiatrist, but it doesn't take one to know she is correct. On several occasions I've seen David on his knees rocking back and forth and crying, 'I wish I could die.' If that is not a psychiatric problem, then I have never seen one."

But the defenders of David's mythology were not easily dissuaded. Dr. South stoutly declared, "I agree with Dr. Wilson. Little David is a happy child every time I see him, and his report cards are good."

Dr. Desmond related the "bizarre" behaviors reported by Jackie and the nurses. "If David becomes psychotic, it is an iatrogenic (illness caused by medical treatment) psychosis brought about by confinement and prolonged deprivation of experience."

Dr. South venomously denounced her and pointed to me, "When you have a patient with a severe psychosis, do you treat the patient by killing him?"

With scarlet face, clinched fists, and strident voice, Dr. Feigin shouted, "I take extreme exception to that remark! Everybody here tries to serve David."

But Dr. South continued, "I resent that a lack of hope has been presented to the family. David's situation is not hopeless. He can be treated."

Dr. Shearer asked on what she based her hope, and a lengthy discussion of treatments and risks ensued. Raphael stared at the ceiling with glazed eyes. Neither Drs. South nor Montgomery commented when Dr. Feigin asked if they wished to have David transferred to their respective institutions for treatment.

Raphael proposed expanding the isolator system and then gradually introducing selected pathogens (germs) in order to see how David would respond.

"No organism is safe for David; his response cannot be predicted!" Dr. Feigin responded angrily. "No research committee will ever give consent." "We did it in Germany with no problem," said Dr. Wilson. Then he directed a supercilious discourse on infections and immunology. I thought the pompous ass is so out of it he doesn't realize he's talking to a renowned expert on infectious diseases!

The Baylor delegate spoke. "It is not unusual for the family of a child with a chronic disease to become attached to the first physicians involved. I suggest a letter be written asking these three to become consultants in providing assistance in David's care." I thought, he's on their side. We're betrayed.

The meeting ended when Dr. Montgomery asked, "How can we help?"

"You can support Dr. Shearer," Dr. Desmond said. She stayed to talk with Drs. South and Montgomery. I walked out with Drs. Shearer and Feigin. We, frustrated and bewildered, just looked at each other. Dr. Shearer shook his head and said, "To a rational, informed outsider we must look like a group of idiots."

A little later, Dr. Feigin came into my office. Neither of us said much. We looked at each other in dismay and wonder. I was consumed with bitterness; he seemed in a state of disbelief. I felt sympathy for him. The poor man hadn't had much experience witnessing the violent emotions David aroused in seemingly rational people.

On December 1, Dr. Desmond, Jackie, and I drove to Lamar Elementary School in Conroe to confer with the psychologist, principal, and the two third-grade teachers on how to normalize David's education and "deinstitutionalize" him. Dr. Coburn and the principal clearly designated our roles as invited consultants. From now on they would be communicating directly with the parents. The Individual Education Plan for David provided more services than required by state law or federal law PL 94-142.

Jackie and I applauded Kathy Jackson's success in forcing David into peer interactions by bringing students to the home. We believed it more important that he associate with peers than with adults. But Kathy expressed frustration. "David remains controlling and refuses to share experiences or his collection of space pictures from NASA with the children," she said. "I consider him more motivated and organized, but he still resists reading."

Dr. Desmond: He needs a library card.

Dr. Coburn: David is a semester above the average of his class, but doesn't have the experiential background of a normal third grader. I wonder if he comprehends what he reads. What can we do to expand his world?

Kathy: I've tried art, songs, poetry, and filmstrips. Then he asks, "Is there a toy store in Taiwan?"

Jackie: The holes in his knowledge impinge on learning. He doesn't know spatial concepts like lake-versus-pond. And, for him, distance is time-based, not linear.

Dr. Coburn: At times his beliefs show up like superstitious knowledge. Jackie: His facility with language convinces people he has great knowledge.

Dr. Coburn: I think we can pull this together with some audio-visual simulations of the oceans, wind, and weather and introduce him to science fiction space books.

Mary: Good luck.

Dr. Desmond answered Kathy's question about the space suit: "We have problems with money." Jackie said the transport allowed him just as much freedom and was safer.

"David hopes the space suit will go away," Dr. Coburn stated.

After discussing how to "fill the holes" in David's knowledge and decrease the thumb sucking and rocking patterns, which were becoming more elaborate and of longer duration, Dr. Coburn declared, "It's a question of responsibility. The parents have a responsibility to their son to alleviate his stress, provide activities, and find resources to assist them with the demands of raising a handicapped child."

"As a team we must help the parents with home stimulation," Jackie said. "The hospital is responsible for both his medical care and environmental milieu."

"We erred in that we did everything except breathe for them," said Dr. Desmond.

Dr. Desmond's anxiety level always soared at any mention of David, but today, being off of her home turf at the hospital, proved especially difficult for her. The next stop was David's house: she intended to look it over and figure out how to rearrange it so he would have "more stimulation." Before we left the hospital, she told us we were not to accept Carol Ann's food. She firmly believed being social with parents diminished the authority and control of the professional. Now, leaving the school, she reiterated her orders and said, "Stop at that restaurant—I'll treat."

At the home, Carol Ann, serving tea and cakes, was obviously hurt by Dr. Desmond's "No thank you, we just ate." Jackie and I visited with David while Dr. Desmond conferred with Carol Ann and her parents.

The drive back proved productive as we came up with ideas to improve David's environment. I suggested overhead lights at home and in the hospital that he could control. Dr. Desmond wanted the wall between his room and the den removed, and the dining room cabinets replaced by a patio door opening to the outside. She felt a flower garden with a birdbath would also be nice.

David returned to the hospital on December 3 and told Donna, "I enjoy being at the hospital. I've been unhappy at home for several years, but I can't tell anyone why—I don't understand it myself. I hope someone is around when I finally figure all this out."

He gave us one glimpse of his home life when he told of worrying about being taken into the den to help decorate the Christmas tree. He said, "I would like to do it, but Dad's way of disconnecting makes me nervous. He takes shortcuts."

David wanted to be the first one to see my doctoral dissertation, so I took it to him straight from the typist. He scrutinized the title page and then silently read the second page: "To David—together we have learned about relentless stress." Tears came to his eyes. "Oh Mary! Thank you." His next statement astounded me. "Now you'll have time to do so many things—travel and go to parties. Will you still have time for me?"

"Of course, love," I assured him.

I continued trying to connect David to the real world as much as possible. Some years before, my son had bought rental property on Westheimer Road in Houston. In one storefront, Bill had a private postal box business.

Now, driving to the airport for his return to Nigeria, he announced, "This packet is for Westheimer. Please take care of it for me. You'll need something to do with school finished." Little did I realize that "Westheimer" would become David's project.

David took over managing the Westheimer property—I explained finances, the laws for eviction, etc. He had fun picking up messages on the post office telephone recorder by remote control. These messages included ones from irate customers who made demands and occasionally cursed. David also returned prospective renters' calls, saying, "Mr. So and So, Mary Murphy, the manager, will speak with you." He, himself, left brief messages for me on the Westheimer message phone: "Please buy a treasure chest for the Beta; don't forget blood in the morning," or "I love you." He phoned on a Sunday morning, "Why did you answer? Hang up so I can leave a message!"

I'd had recurring problems with my feet and had had surgery twice. Now a bump appeared on the top of my left foot and, if I hit it against anything, the pain lasted a long time. David's TV stand, fabricated from stainless steel tubing, had two rough, protruding braces which I invariably hit when I squeezed by the TV to the window. One evening David, pointing to padding surrounded by yellow tape on the braces, said, "Mary how do you like that?" To everyone's comment on what looked like giant turkey drumsticks, he stated, "I had to have that done for Mary."

David grieved over Donna's leaving and angrily accused, "Somebody else will take my place with you!" She promised to visit and call often.

Jackie and the nurses reported disturbing behaviors—withdrawal and silent mouthing of words. David unnerved the dental hygienist by graphically describing various ways to kill birds and then "drifting off into another world."

At the December 16, 1980, CDP meeting Dr. Desmond summarized the school conference and informed the parents, "David is often bored and is not learning enough to satisfy his active mind."

How painful it was to listen to the parents relate their futile attempts to engage their son in activities and conversation. Carol Ann confessed, "Except for an occasional card game, I have been unable to 'play' with him since he was five."

David Sr. said, "About all I can do is to demonstrate fishing gear."

Lynn read the list of proposed environment improvements—lights, etc. Carol Ann said, "A sliding patio door would expose David to spectators. We were told we had to hide him. Has that changed?" David Sr. questioned if it would be possible to put a microwave oven in, and if a room similar to a domed swimming pool cover could be sterilized. Dr. Shearer said no to both.

David Sr. stated that his son needed more complicated, sophisticated toys. I showed a miniature tool kit, agreeing that David "needs screwdrivers." David Sr. examined the set and commented, "I'd like my son to have this, and I'd like one of these for myself."

"I have another set you can have," I told him.

After much persuasion it was decided the tool set could go in.

Carol Ann asked, "Then, can an Erector set go in? I bought one last Christmas and was told no."

"He has the judgment to handle an Erector set," I said. David Sr. smiled. Dr. Desmond brought up questions of responsibility if potentially dangerous toys went in the isolator. "Remember, he jabbed holes with a spoon."

David's exit from the hospital on December 18, before the Christmas holidays, was early in the morning and swift. Donna followed the van so there was no wait for him, missing his mother.

Right before Christmas, the local volunteer fire department made David an honorary member. He grumbled, "Just because I have to live with all this bubble doesn't mean I want to be treated differently. I don't want to be treated as if I'm special." He abided by his mother's order to be polite, but initiated no conversation with the firefighters.

Meanwhile, with my dissertation done, I was free for the first time in ages. I slept ten to twelve hours a night, but still looked exhausted. During my physical examination, I told William Obenour, M.D., "I'm caught up on my sleep but look at my eyes."

"I know just the right plastic surgeon for you," he said with a smile. I decided to have the surgery done as a treat to myself.

The herculean struggle to keep the isolator system working never stopped—the carpenters ingeniously kept the ports reinforced.

Lynn and I partially solved some of the creasing of the crib by equalizing the stress. We directed that two metal rods, three-eighths of an inch in diameter, be run through channels glued to the top of the bubble. Four giant rubber bands were knotted to the ends of the rods and attached to ceiling springs.

Similarly, shoring up David's deteriorating psyche was an ongoing task but palliative measures were not so easy or obvious. Lynn, feeling pressured by David's emotional state, told Dr. Shearer she needed assistance in dealing with the psychological aspects of David's care.

On January 6, 1981, David yelled at Lynn, "Get out of this house! Leave me alone!" She and Carol Ann tried to halt the violent tantrum by encouraging him to talk.

After letting Lynn hold him, he quieted, but refused to be specific about the trouble: "If I decide to tell anyone what upset me, you and Mom will be the first to know." It was apparent that he had been set off by his frustrations regarding the intercom, which he used to hear his teacher. He did not always hear the teacher and could not talk unless she released her button. She needed a remote control, he needed an interject button. For the next three months, the school phone connection resulted in a series of screaming fits.

At the January 13, 1981, CDP meeting, we discussed David's interactions with other people:

Mary: He didn't interact well when he was an infant.

Desmond: Yes, he did. I saw him weekly. He was a vigorous, active baby. Mary: At one year of age, people talking to or at him, never with him, created problems.

Jackie: That's still true. It's exactly like when we visited the home and saw the grandmother's concept of his difference. She thinks of him as completely separate from her other grandchildren. She said, "I admire the way you two find it so easy to talk to David. When I stand there, I don't talk—I can't—and it makes me cry."

Desmond: Let's defer that. I want to discuss the stresses on and of the team. The visit to his home triggered my worst stress. Our stresses interfere with our professional efficiency. We need help.

Lynn:	Yes, I've been really frustrated by David's emotional outbursts over trivial matters. He gets completely hysterical. I try to get him to talk but he won't answer.
Dr. Shearer:	Give us a specific instance.
Lynn:	Well, the time I mentioned about the intercom to school, and the time when his mother inadvertently threw his last pair of blue jeans in the trash. When we got there, he was wrapped in a blanket, and we didn't know what was wrong. How do we manage?
Shearer:	What was his mother's reaction?
Lynn:	She was angry and told him there was no reason to get so upset about such little things.
Shearer:	How is she coping?
Lynn:	She says okay, but she sure looks tired.
Susan:	Well, it is kind of terrible for a nine-year-old boy to lose his last pair of pants.
Jackie:	Yes, any other boy can go to the laundry hamper and get a dirty pair.
Mary:	He is more open with his anger now.
Jackie:	At this age, kids get angry with their mother and for him; it's the pits—double jeopardy. He can't say it. He can't get out or do anything constructive. It's the devil if he does, and the devil if he doesn't.
Lynn:	His mother seems to be recognizing an emotional problem.
Shearer:	The question is, can the people here still help David? Jackie, do you think you can still help him, or is it diminishing returns?
Jackie:	I'm afraid I'm reaching diminished returns. I am reluctant to cut back on the time. He depends on it. I cannot and will not abandon him, but I'm frustrated, and I don't know where to go. I can't see that I'm making any big change in his behavior. A sounding board and assistance for myself would be good. I have no illusions that the meetings are going to be magic or change anything, but they might get us from day one to day two. We need something to keep us from burning out. I don't want to stop seeing him, especially now with his level of

cognitive development. It is difficult to know what is going on in his head. He asks questions. It is difficult to answer them with honesty and compassion.

For example, what do you say when he asks, "Why do I go to school?" In David's case honesty has to be tempered, and somebody, an outsider, could give us some guidelines and ferret out what's been told to him and know what the discrepancies are. He has a problem with trust.

Susan: It is difficult working with someone who answers your questions with questions.

Lynn: I know, he questions me about all our meetings—he's testing me.

What about the answers to his questions?

Shearer: You don't lie.

Lynn: I've avoided questions but haven't told him a lie. Susan: Does he question you, Dr. Shearer?

Shearer: I don't see him very much. I don't want to be enmeshed like the former doctors, so I avoid spending any time with him.

Lynn: He wants to know why all the changes—the house and schedule.

Mary: We see his rage coming out.

Desmond: Maybe he needs the punching bag we discussed.

Jackie: He doesn't have any physical separation from his parents or individuation from adults. He's angry with his mother; therefore, he's angry with himself and pounds on himself. Lately he has been hitting himself so much.

Shearer: Dr. Hansen has been counseling the team. He's now involved in the diagnostic part and is the expert on David's mental status. If he continues in a diminished capacity as a consultant, we may be asking too much of him. Should we go outside for someone else?

Desmond: We're in a limbo situation.

Mary: All of you are now where I was over two… three years ago.

Desmond: Could we get help through Dr. Hansen's group?

Betty:	I am uncomfortable talking about Carol Ann when Dr. Hansen's in the meeting.
Mary:	Did you have anybody in mind?
Shearer:	Dr. Jay Tamow.
Jackie:	He is really good in case conferences. When the meeting is over, you know all the issues.
Dr. Shearer:	We've got to touch on the space suit. It will be ready in three months. I refuse to take responsibility for that machine. I met with them; they didn't like hearing it's a bother, and David hates it. Some time ago, someone should have said there is no point. After a $100,000 investment they want something back. They have a right to be angry.
Mary:	NASA has been getting double messages, one from us, and the other from the parents.
Lynn:	I talked with the microbiologist and he seems to want to drop the project.
Dr. Shearer:	Searching out the impracticability would be the avenue to take.

The meeting adjourned.

On Thursday, January 29, 1981, David said, "Look at this finger—it's worn out from dialing your number. It's almost seven-thirty, Mary. I was so afraid you didn't know I was back. Where were you?"

"The spa with Carolyn Grimmett."

"You parked in the doctor's lot? You really are a doctor, aren't you? Well, if you don't mind, I'll still call you Mary. Now, tell me the latest in the Westheimer file, but first let me pick up the post office messages."

David's first night back always entailed cleaning the fishbowls, a grubby job I attempted to lighten by buying an aquarium with a filter. He would have no part of it—he liked the bowls. As I labored at the sink in the anteroom, Dr. Larry Tabor stood in the door and commented, "You must be the highest paid fishbowl cleaner in the world."

I retorted, "What pay?" Of the thousands of hours I spent with David over his lifetime, none of it was part of my official schedule. It was on my own time.

The next evening David inquired, "Are you getting a handle on the new Mary? Well, I don't think you can do much about your hair. Don't change too much—I like the way you are now. Go to the spa right after work so you can be here on time. Remember, you promised to come every night—we only have two weeks."

The two weeks were not pleasant. He was irascible, and one thing after another kept him in an uproar. First, Betty, his backup nurse who played beautifully with him, told him she was leaving. Then an extra blood drawing was required because the lab "misplaced" his blood.

Along with worries caused by David's own temper were the intrusions of curiosity seekers. Saturday night, a couple barged in and frightened him by pushing on the bubble and demanding, "Why is that boy in a balloon? We saw him from the street and came for a better look." Earlier I had seen them stroll down the hall and had called security. I shoved them back and reprimanded, "Three times you came through a door with NO ADMITTANCE! Security is on their way!"

David's safety from outsiders was a never-ending worry. Some letters from deranged or fanatic people made my hair stand on end—violent threats because we "imprisoned a healthy boy" or refused their "sure cure."

Sunday afternoon, my mother called. She was certain Susie, her dog, was dying. Renee, her brothers, and I sat in the living room as Susie peacefully died on my mother's lap. I called David to say I would be late. When I arrived, he asked me "Why have you been crying?"

"Susie died."

"Why didn't you stop it—why didn't you do something?"

"I couldn't. She was eighteen years old; that's very old for a dog. She didn't suffer. She was tired and worn out."

His ongoing fascination with death kept the questions coming: "Did your mother and Renee cry hard? Tell me where and how you buried her." I answered patiently.

Minutes before the February 10 CDP meeting, Carol Ann gave me a story written by David for a class assignment. She said it moved her and all of the school people to tears. It had the same effect on me:

MY BEST FRIEND

I have a friend her name is Mary Murphy. She and I have great times together. But one time I was really happy was when she bought me my first fish. But what really makes her really special is the care she gives me and the way she loves me. And we play hide and go seek a lot too. She comes every other night and parks her car out front of the hospital. She tells me stories about herself. I think Mary is a very nice person and I love her.

—David

At the meeting, Dr. Shearer introduced Jay Tarnow, M.D., and said, "Lynn can tell us some of the problems."

Lynn: I would like to know how to handle the outbursts…

Jackie: I share Lynn's concern. You can't help him physically; you have to encourage him verbally. I feel helpless. In reality, we can't help him.

More discussion ensued about David's behaviors and the team's frustrations.

Tarnow: Just what are your hopes and fantasies about how I can assist you?

Shearer: I see your role not as a therapist with David, but to help us. The team needs help.

Desmond: We want to know how best to serve David. I'm concerned about the holes in his knowledge. The lack of experience makes David's education more difficult.

Jackie: It's a great concern of many, and I expect that as he progresses along in the grades, the gaps in experience will reveal themselves more and more. Experience is the base for abstract reasoning. He doesn't know how to cope because of his lack of knowledge and understanding. I feel helpless with no answers. I feel there can be a solution. What I need is a day-to-day, objective sounding board.

Shearer: This committee meets each month and discusses new things and practical matters. We listen and respond as best we can to the needs of all.

There followed a discussion of the space suit. I pointed out, once again, that David had extracted a promise from me to avoid pushing him on getting into the suit.

Tarnow: I'm in awe—What a relationship you have with him. Does David know about these meetings?

Mary: Yes, he usually knows everything that goes on. He asks different participants questions, pieces things together, and he's intuitive. He looks at faces and eyes and notices things that most others wouldn't.

Jackie: Yes, he has had eye-to-eye contact with adults all of his life because of the way the bubble is placed.

Desmond: One of the things we're concerned with is that he has no way to release his feelings.

Mary: David asked me what other boys do when they're angry and why he does the things he does. I've told him it's because when other boys are upset or things go wrong they can run out or slam a door, etc.

Tarnow: Mary, you are his therapist.

Shearer: No, she is not his therapist. He has not had therapy. Dr. Hansen did specifically recommend therapy, but it has not been carried out.

Mary: I don't know exactly how to describe my role. It changes. When he was three, I was brought in to get him to go into the playroom, and then it just evolved. It was like getting caught in a giant whirlpool; once in, there's no way back.

Tarnow: Apparently you have a very special relationship with this child. Carol Ann, how do you feel about this?

Carol Ann: I think they have a unique relationship, and it's a very comforting one for me. I know that when he is at the hospital, she gives him the care and attention that I would give him. I have been very comfortable with her role with him.

Tarnow: Does your husband come?

Carol Ann: No. He refuses. He says he has no problems and doesn't need help. Little David, above all, minds and respects his father.

That evening, David asked, "Did you like my story? Was I born with a good brain—a better one than those kids you see?"

"Yes, love. Yes to both. It's beautiful."

"Jackie and Shawn are good friends, too, almost as good as you. You're number one. When I'm at the hospital, Jackie's number two, and when I'm home, Shawn is number two."

Shawn was David's one and only peer friend.

David referred to himself as *Encyclopedia David*. He had always been fascinated with words and asked me to define unknown ones, but if a controversy arose or I did not know a word, we used the dictionary.

Upon this return to the hospital, his list of unknown words included "incest" and "homosexual." A brief explanation sufficed for incest—relatives marrying.

He had heard "homosexual" sometime before on the TV show *All in the Family* and accepted that it described the relationship of two men living together. Then came his specific questions: "Is gay and homosexual the same?" and "Just what is homosexual?"

"Aside from friendship," I said, "There are two types of intimate adult relationships—heterosexual and homosexual. The most common and most accepted is heterosexual—partners of the opposite sex, a man and a woman. Homosexuals prefer their life partner to be their own sex."

That same week, we watched two men "marry" on a TV show, and read a newspaper article on homosexual legislation. The controversy surrounding homosexuality amazed David. "Why does everybody get so upset when two men want to marry each other? What difference does it make? Why should anybody care? If two men want to live together or two women want to live together, why isn't that okay?"

"In our culture," I said, "The main reason people marry is to have children. If a man marries a man, or a woman a woman, there can be no children."

"Well, that makes sense," he conceded.

His interest in homosexuality continued because of the daily local newscasts on the infamous Montrose community, Houston's gay area. The Westheimer property that David helped me to manage was in the middle of the area.

Later, more sensational and more intriguing to David was AIDS. In those early days of the epidemic, he pointed out the seriousness of AIDS to me and prophesied that it would spread to other groups. The combination of the similarity between congenital immune deficiency and the acquired immune deficiency as well as the gay involvement made AIDS infinitely fascinating to him.

On Thursday afternoon, Jackie spent time with David while preparations for going home were made. Cheerful and talkative, he told her, "I really like this transport, especially when it's all packed with my toys. At home, I sleep in here even though my mom and dad think it's stupid. I have everything in here to survive—even a balanced snack."

Friday morning, after waiting an hour for Carol Ann, he greeted her with, "Miss Late Bird, as usual."

He pleaded for me to ride home with him. "My schedule—I can't." As we started down the hall, he sent me back for something and remarked, "It's so nice to look at you from a distance."

Two guards took us through the hall, which was filled with people pointing and staring.

Both my plastic and orthopedic surgeries were scheduled for the same day, during the first week of March 1981. Knowing that the thought of a surgeon's knife assaulting my eyes would panic David, I called Carol Ann. We agreed that we would tell him only about the foot surgery. She then relayed David's orders, "Have a spinal so you can watch—I want all the details."

A week after the surgery, I phoned Carol Ann. "I've never been so pleased with anything—my eyes are wonderful."

"I'm glad you had the surgery—you sound like your old self again." "What do you mean?"

"The surgery must have done something for you. Big David and I have discussed the change in you, we wondered what had happened—if something had gone wrong in your life."

"No, just work, finishing school, and everything."

"I know the dissertation took a lot of time, and we consider it a great honor that you dedicated it to our son. We felt something other than work happened."

"Frankly, I have been exhausted physically and mentally since last summer."

"Oh, what happened last summer?"

"The shock of being told that decisions had to be made about David's future paralyzed me. He's not my son, my feelings could never be as deep as yours, but he means a lot to me."

"I know you love him. Believe me, I thank God every day that you do care. No matter what, you never neglect my son."

"I can't cope with indecision. Your postponing talking to your husband drove me up the wall."

"My style is just the opposite of yours. I have to think things over in my mind for a long time before I make a decision or discuss it with my husband."

"In David's case, indecision was, for me, intolerable. The past year was exhausting."

"I understand and am really glad to know that nothing happened to you. I have not given up hope."

15.

RESIGNATION AND DESPAIR

"Mary, you look tired," David said. "It's been over six weeks since we slept all night. Right? Maybe you need eye surgery again. Remember you were disappointed when I didn't notice you had surgery on your eyes? But, I did say you looked pretty."

"Certainly I remember rushing up to your room the minute you arrived so you and your mother could admire my eyes. You said, 'Put a foot up here.'"

The afternoon of Friday, March 20, 1981, David's interest was indeed in my feet.

"I see where he cut and stitched. Does it hurt?"

"A little," I said. "Look at my face. I had cosmetic surgery." "How did he take the bumps off your feet?"

"My feet were propped up, and after he made the incision, the nurse handed him a silver chisel and hammer. I said, 'Surely you're not going to use those on my feet?'"

David roared with laughter. "Well, surely he would use a hammer and chisel to knock them off. What did you expect? I'm going to tell everybody!"

"Look at my face and listen. After Dr. Siff finished, Dr. Gerow did my eyes. I was in a twilight zone from Valium."

"You aren't joking. Come closer. I don't see stitch marks." "I'm thrilled with the surgery, but no one notices. I thought you would."

"Did the anesthetic make you sick?"

"Yes, I vomited all night, and my back hurt because they wouldn't let me turn over. Louise stayed with me."

He probed for more morbid details of the nausea. I was a little disappointed, but I suppose that depth of interest or compassion is about all one could expect from a nine-year-old boy. Carol Ann thought I looked great.

That evening, David, rather subdued, remained quiet. I sensed a change—a puzzling one. Had some type of resignation set in? I remarked, "You're different. Have you settled something in your mind? Has something happened?"

"It's just your imagination. I know you are sad that I have to live in a bubble, but I am not sad about it because I have never been out, and I haven't known another way to live."

Sunday evening, one of his shrimp disappeared. I found it on the floor all dried up. He insisted, "Put him in the bowl. Maybe he's not really dead." Incredibly, David's instinct had been correct: in a few minutes the shrimp swam around.

David looked me straight in the eyes. "You told me there was no in-between—you were either dead or alive. That shrimp was in-between. Explain that."

I didn't have a clue, but suggested, "I think maybe freshwater shrimp had to learn to adapt to no water when the sun evaporated their ponds. They lay in dry sand until it rained. Maybe that's what happened to this one."

Tuesday afternoon Jackie reported that David was withdrawn and refused to engage in any activities. He told her, "Don't look at the fishbowl right now because one of my fish is going to the bathroom and doesn't want everyone to see."

That evening he asked me, "What kind of kids did you see today?" After I described several to him, he commented, "Well, everybody's born with a problem. You've got your feet and me—look at this mess I've got. But yours is worse—I don't hurt and your feet do."

Wednesday at noon I took my new colleague, Judy Rozelle, to meet David. She immediately became a friend—a helpful friend.

Thursday afternoon Jackie found David quiet and pensive, though he would not identify why. He sat, rocking and sucking his thumb, or stood, sucking his thumb and pounding his penis. She could not engage him in any activity, but he questioned her about pets that she had owned that had subsequently died—he wanted to be assured they had received a "proper burial."

That evening he asked me if I ever saw boys with Duchene muscular dystrophy.

"Sometimes. It is a terrible degenerative disease...."

"I know that from TV. The genetics is what I want to know. Boys inherit it from mothers."

"It's X-linked recessive transmission; the defective gene carried by the female is expressed in her male children. The probability is a flip of a coin. A boy born to a carrier has a fifty-fifty chance of having the disease, and each girl has a fifty-fifty chance of being a carrier."

"I know all that. How do the chromosomes work?"

"Humans have forty-six chromosomes, actually twenty-three pairs. At conception, twenty-three in the sperm combine with twenty-three in the egg to form a zygote that grows into a baby.

"Twenty-two pairs are autosomal and one pair is the sex chromosome—girls have two Xs and boys have an X and a Y. It's a fifty-fifty chance of being a boy or a girl. The zygote gets one X from the mother and either an X or a Y from the father. If one of the mother's X chromosomes has a defective gene, the baby will have a fifty-fifty chance of getting either the good or the bad X. If a girl gets the bad X, she'll be a carrier because she has a good X from the father for counterbalance. If a boy gets the bad X, he won't have a good X partner. He's XY, so he'll have the disease."

"What happens to the children of the males?"

"If he has a good X, his children will be healthy. If he has a bad X and, therefore, the disease, all his daughters will inherit his bad X and be carriers, but the sons will be okay."

The next day, he asked, "What is wrong with the baby girl from Dallas who has dozens of relatives wandering around CRC?" A baby girl with SCID was now being treated; the staff had decided not to tell David about it, in case she did poorly. Because he asked, however, I did not lie to him.

"She has no immune system."

"Oh, that's why they won't mention her and gown up before they go in her room. Let's go over the X-linked genes again. Okay, SCID is X-linked recessive, right?"

"Yes."

"Well, then, what about that baby SCID girl?"

"There is more than one type of immune deficiency. I'm not a geneticist, but her case has to be either an autosomal recessive or dominate type of transmission. The defective gene is on one of the twenty-two autosomal chromosomes, so it isn't sex linked."

"Oh, I understand. "There was a long silence; he seemed to be mulling the implications of everything I had told him. Finally, he said, "I know you are sad because I am in this bubble, but I'm not. It's all I know. But I know you must be sad."

David's curiosity was boundless. Pretty, tiny premature twins on CRC intrigued him and prompted many questions about the birth process. Then he announced, "We are going to discuss the facts of life." I gave simple, factual answers to each of his specific questions, but when we really got into the nitty-gritty of it all, he yelped. "Oh! God! Mary! Stop! I don't want to hear any more!"

Just then came sheer excitement—an explosion on Fannin Street. A car jumped the curb, hit a lamppost and knocked over a gas tank. Watching with morbid glee, hoping the tank would explode, he mused—"How big will the explosion be? It wouldn't be enough to break my windows would it? "Wonderful, wonderful bustling activities soon followed—an ambulance, police cars, two fire trucks, and a hoard of wreckers. The commotion over, he said, "That's the most exciting thing that ever happened! Go down there and read any writing on the tank."

On Monday all he could talk about was the news reports about the attempted assassination of President Reagan. "Why would anybody do that?" Jackie, thank goodness, saw him before I did and answered his questions. It was tough for adults across the country to explain it to their children, but it was a particular challenge to explain psychopathic behavior to a child who had never even witnessed an argument.

The blood drawing on Friday had gone fine, so had the one on Tuesday morning. I was proud of myself. I did not become nauseated. That evening,

David asked, "Can you come in the morning? Blood again. Let me tell you I am angry—an extra blood drawing."

The next morning went terribly. For one thing, both David's arms were sore. After they inserted the needle, he drew back and had to be stuck again. When he started perspiring and trembling, the nurses moved away so I could calm him.

"My arm's so sore. I'm going to faint. I don't trust them." I held him until he settled down.

"We'll try one more time and that's it."

"The lab will make us, Dr. Shearer will make us do it. I'm so afraid I'm losing control of my mind."

"Listen, a sore arm and being stuck with a needle have nothing to do with losing your mind. We're going to try one more time, and if that doesn't work, I will tell Dr. Shearer no more—two days in a row is too much."

"What if he says we have to?"

"I'll go to Dr. Feigin. Come on now; let's get this over. I must get back to work. I'll eat lunch with you. Now take a deep breath, then call the nurses." He smiled and three minutes later the blood was in the tubes.

Wednesday, April 1, was Potts' birthday. I went up to celebrate at her party, but she wanted to talk: "At times I can't face David. I look at him, and I'm afraid I'll cry. I can't talk about the Astros." (Potts and David had a ritual. She asked, "What will we do when you get out?" He replied, "Go to an Astros game and have a hamburger, French fries, and a Coke.")

Potts, in a chronic state of consternation over David's not eating, encouraged him to at least drink more water. She thought perhaps he perspired a lot at home since the house was rather warm. Whatever she worked on, she had me working on, too, so I pushed water. She also found some germ-free water packed tuna, which he liked. In the past year, he had grown an inch-and-a-half taller, to fifty-one-and-three-eighths inches and was up to fifty-six pounds, a gain of seven pounds. He was still very slim. His weight remained at, or below, the fifth percentile—in other words, ninety-five boys out of one hundred weighed more at his age. His height consistently stayed at the twenty-fifth percentile.

David became obsessed with the hunger strike of the protesters in Ireland. Question after question: "Why? Do they suffer?" Once during such a conversation with Jackie, he stated, "I'm very hungry." He asked if it was okay if he started on dinner and proceeded hungrily to consume a jar of meat sticks. When, later, he threatened to go on a hunger strike, Jackie and I were concerned. Getting him to eat had always been a trial; we knew he could easily quit eating. In private, I expressed my worry to Dr. Hansen. He smiled and advised, "Let the boy have his fantasies."

For weeks David had blamed the female Beta fish for all his problems—anything that went wrong was her fault. The night before David went home, he said, "I don't want to hurt your feelings, but would you please take the female Beta home with you? Transfer her to the big bowl and clean everything inside real good and make sure the pink valentine heart stays on the bowl. I'm going to fix the bowl perfect."

He carefully arranged everything on the purple rocks. I started to pour water back in the bowl, but he yelled "No! She stays in the big bowl. Print FOR RENT and tape it on one of those toothpicks in your purse. You know, I've been starving her for a long time."

Her demise was quick. He never inquired.

The next morning, April 4, I arrived very early because I had to test a child at 8:15. I left David's room promising to return to say goodbye.

Later, when the nurses started to cap off the transport, he had an anxiety attack—he perspired, hyperventilated, and held his breath. Jackie and Lynn, both alarmed, settled him down by saying they would wait for me before disconnecting him. Lynn called Mildred to tell me to hurry. When I arrived, he fretfully whimpered, "My stomach hurts. Read me the *Wall Street Journal.*"

Carol Ann arrived and told about some Easter chicks she had acquired: "Everything I have survives," she commented. Jackie turned white. As we left CRC, David said, "I'll drink three bottles of water each day, and you drink eight glasses full—you're old." While we loaded him in the van, he sobbed, "I love you, I love you, I love you. Please come see me!"

"I will." I did.

A week after David went home, I wrote in his chart, "I have decided that some type of resignation, not despair, has set in. He is working hard to conform and be a good boy at an extreme emotional cost. I am more concerned at this point than ever before."

In April 1981, Dr. Shearer decided to discharge David from TCH. Beginning the first of August, he would live at home for six months and return to the hospital for just a one-week stay in December and again in July. The parents were to be responsible for routine isolator care, picking up weekly supplies from TCH, and putting them in the isolator. The hospital would furnish and maintain the isolators, provide the food and all supplies except clothes and toys, pack and sterilize the supplies, take cultures for NASA, and medically monitor David.

On May 8, 1981, Drs. Shearer and Desmond met with the parents to inform them of the new schedule and to discuss the latest research in immunology, which held no promise for a treatment. It was agreed that Carol Ann would tell David of the new schedule.

Jackie and I were devastated. David had yet to adjust to the six-weeks-at-home, two-at-the-hospital schedule and relied so heavily upon us for support. To be honest, we worried about actual neglect. It was humanly impossible for Carol Ann, or anyone, to cope with him and the bubbles for six whole months. Anyone staying with David had to be trained and willing to assume the colossal responsibility of keeping the isolators going. David Sr. worked every day. Their neighbor, Raymond Aust, knew the mechanics of the isolator system, and Raymond's wife, Doris, and a host of friends would help. But still, the thought of being cooped up with David day in and day out without relief for six months boggled Jackie's and my mind.

On Thursday, May 14, David and six classmates put on a play. The invitations read: "We would like to invite you to THE PUPPET SHOW, Starring Doubt, Hate, Spite and Love." Jackie, Lynn, and I went to see it.

The playwright, David, knew little of travel and places; his story reflected life as he knew it and contained endearing sentimentality: A group of bickering children, traveling by train to a summer vacation at the beach, argue until Love walks in. At the end, the children are happy friends and sing "The Rainbow Connection." Carol Ann served a buffet, and we all had a wonderful time.

The next day, when David returned to the hospital, he was busy writing a "secret play." I visited late Saturday afternoon because I had a date that night. Sunday, I spent four hours with him and then went to a party. Monday, he stated, "I made it okay last night, but Saturday night without you was lonely. Afternoons don't count. Promise you'll never miss two nights in a row again."

"I promise. I haven't had time for parties. My mother says at my age I should take all opportunities."

He remarked, "She can say that again."

Tuesday evening, when I arrived early, he asked, "When is that bastard" (meaning my date) "leaving town?" After I left, he saw a roach, demanded it be destroyed and refused to go to sleep until the nurses produced the roach—dead. By now he had a full-blown bug phobia—bugs, to him, were giant germs.

Saturday night, David asked, "If you had three wishes what would they be?"

"You could probably guess at least two of them."

"Mary, I don't want out of the bubble. What I want you to do is to go on roach patrol. We've got to make sure there are no roaches around here." I folded a magazine and turned the lights off. We sat in the dark, talking and watching the stars for ten minutes. To his "Ready," I stood poised with my weapon, ready to kill roaches, when he pulled the overhead light on. There were none.

Bill called at the crack of dawn. "Mother, I have a little problem. I'm in Amsterdam with Akuu—I couldn't leave him in Kaduna. Call the U.S. veterinary to get his approval. I have everything required. If you can't get it worked out, I'll fly on to Mexico City and try for entry through Florida. Call me back."

I went to David's room very early so he could be in on the calls. The vet, for a fee, agreed to meet me at the airport custom's office at ten o'clock that night. The friendly vet told me that no bird was more beautiful or intelligent than an African Grey. If the parrot passed his inspection, he would give a special dispensation, but Akuu would have to be flown to El Paso for a thirty-day quarantine. Everything was set, but the KLM satellite was down. Within a few minutes KLM called, "Mr. Dunlap is traveling with two parrots."

David questioned, "Two?" KLM repeated, "Two parrots."

That evening before I left for the airport, David warned, "Bill doesn't know we arranged everything. He might be asleep and not get off the plane. Then what?"

"Ridiculous."

"We'll see."

The customs office provided hours of conversation with David—the things people tried to bring in. The vet held up a jar with a piece of fruit covered with worms—"fruit fly larvae." The KLM supervisor and a man carrying the birds walked in. The vet examined the "gorgeous birds." The customs man asked, "Where is Mr. Dunlap?" No one knew the supervisor went to check and returned with a sleepy Bill, "Mother, I was going on to Mexico."

"Why didn't you tell me there were two birds?"

"Mother, I have faith. If you could get one in, you could get two in." The KLM man and the vet had to witness the parrots loaded on the plane to

El Paso. The vet assured us that the vet in El Paso was a kind, competent man and gave me the phone number.

David, of course, said, "I told you." We called El Paso. The birds were fine but had problems with the Interior Department.

The vet in El Paso assured us everything was in order and under no circumstances would he release the birds.

David summed the cost and said, "Who would believe anything about this whole deal?"

I usually waited for David to introduce a topic or ask questions before launching into a serious or profound discussion because the teachers and nurses were vexed and justly concerned about his accelerating penis pounding.

But, I decided we needed to talk. "You once asked me to define masturbation. It's time for us to discuss it in detail. The way you pound yourself is considered a form of masturbation. It is a taboo subject and many people believe it a vile habit. But kids in every culture masturbate; it's universal. In psychology, it's considered a normal phase of development—a way to release tension."

"I'm with you. Go on."

"Masturbation can be a terrible habit if it's done too much. Some people have strange ideas—masturbating makes you insane or gives you pimples. The real problem is, if excessive then it leads to guilt and self-devaluation.

"A kid resolves to never again do the forbidden act, but the urges take over and he does, and then he feels like hell for being weak. Your father forbids thumb sucking, but you do it without thinking. The same can happen with masturbation. Doing it in public means trouble."

"I hear you. Thank you."

David's leaving for home on the twenty-ninth of May was uneventful. Carol Ann reported that she felt he had accepted the idea of staying more or less permanently at home, beginning in August, and that she herself was feeling more positive about the change.

Lynn, after visiting the home twice, told me that David had remarked several times that he needed to discuss something with me. I visited him briefly on the afternoon of his return to the hospital, July 10. Agitated and distant, he stated, "I have a problem to discuss tonight." But that evening, he refused to discuss the problem, and lapsed into more rocking, thumb sucking, and penis pounding.

The next evening, determined not to let David forestall again, I said, "I know it's difficult to talk about feelings and problems, but we must talk."

"Yes, Mary, it is hard for me to talk about my problem. Promise not to tell anyone. How can I tell my mother that I don't want to live at home? I love my parents very much, but I can't tolerate the thought of six months. I don't want to go home ever. It's being caged in a dark and dreary house, surrounded by nothing. We have to find a way out of this mess." He had often heard me use the phrase, where there's a will, there's a way, and now he said, "I've got the will, now you have to find the way out."

David paced, threw himself down, pounded his fists, screamed and cursed with such venom that I wanted to run, to scream for help. After more than an hour of vitriolic tirade, he resumed talking. "You gotta thin brain. Whose decision was this anyway and when did you know?"

"The decision was made in April; no one person made it. It's the right decision. You should be with your parents and school friends. A hospital is no place for a boy to grow up. Medically your hospital stays can't be justified; you're not sick. I have no power to change the schedule, and even if I did, I wouldn't. Believe me, it is for the best. Love, I do understand you do not want to go six months without a change. You would be more upset with a two-week-home and six-month-hospital schedule. Look, let's take it one day at a time. You can control how you deal with this."

"Why didn't they do something to me before I was old enough to care? I have thought about the choices. Now it's too late for me to get out because I don't know what will happen—I can't handle not knowing. Maybe before I could have, but not now. They should have done something when I was three.

When I was three I wouldn't have cared. When all this mess started nine years ago, didn't they ever think about or realize that they were dealing with a life, my life? They made decisions without ever thinking about anything except what they wanted to do; not about all this crap I'm in, and now they make decisions because of money—not caring about my feelings."

"That's not true, we all care about you and your feelings. Money is not the issue. Money to maintain you is a problem, but no one here will ever let money come before you. Believe me, Drs. Feigin and Shearer are trying to do what is best for you; remember, they didn't put you in isolation."

"I am a mouse surrounded by ten cats, and there are no dogs to chase the cats away. The worst feeling about being caged in this damn crap and shit is that I feel so helpless. It is so awful to feel helpless—awful—awful—helpless! (A storm of collected grievances against the original doctors poured out with raucous profanity.) What am I going to do? You've got chicken shit for a brain! I'm surprised that you have enough brain to get out of bed and get dressed each morning!

"What I need is a plan so I can stay here longer—what's more, you be ready with one in three weeks. When they first told me about the six months, I decided to slash the sleep isolator when Shawn was there so he could cap off the supply while I rushed into the playroom. Then I figured that would only be temporary, at most a few days back at the hospital for repairs. Then I thought about burning down the house, but couldn't figure out how to do it without me and the bubble going up in flames. Hell, if everything burned down, that would settle it. I'll tell you one thing—those three doctors that started all this mess haven't been around lately. Where do you suppose I could get some legal advice?"

"A lawyer."

"Preposterous, me call a lawyer! What lawyer would talk to a nine-year-old in the fourth grade?" he howled, laughing. "Well, I'm helpless. Mother is helpless. You are powerless. As a matter of fact, everyone that has anything to do with this mess is helpless. Yes, everyone is helpless except me. I've got a good brain, and I'm the only one in this goddamn mess who's not helpless. Gee, it sure did feel good to talk and get this all off my chest. Poor Mary, I dump all my shit on you. You look tired, let's play your favorite game, hide-and-go-seek."

On Monday evening, David again brought up his quandary: "I'm the only one in this mess that can make a decision, and I've decided the only solution is to come out. We both know I can't survive. Dying doesn't worry me. Not knowing what will happen to me is the problem—I can't stand not knowing. Mary, what could we expect? Don't answer—you don't know. I need to know exactly what will Dr. Shearer do? Will I be in a room like the SCID babies and everybody will have to gown up? Will I be sick a long time? He'll probably give me gamma globulin. How did he plan to do it last summer? God, all the questions. I must have answers before I decide, and he's the only one who has any answers. Trouble is, he doesn't believe children have the right to make decisions. I feel I've some right to make a decision about my life because no one else can or will. My case is different. Maybe he will listen."

"I think he would talk with you."

"Would you please make the arrangements? But first promise two things: don't tell him what I want to discuss, and promise you will be here, too."

When I told David that Dr. Shearer would meet with him Friday at noon, he demanded reassurance that I had not told Shearer why. He then started working on his script for the encounter. David's moods over the next few days ranged from joking and pleasant to agitated and withdrawn.

Thursday, near midnight, David phoned to practice: "Dr. Shearer, I want to discuss a serious matter. I would like some medical information about my case. I know you can't give me exact answers, but what could I expect if I came out?" The next morning he rehearsed as I drank coffee. He was relieved that my schedule was unchanged and feeling confident that he was prepared.

At noon, I stood by the playroom to avoid interfering; David's back was to me. Dr. Shearer stood between the window and TV, facing me. David politely invited him to sit on the stool. Shearer said he preferred to stand. With bravado, David ordered, "Sit down!"

Shearer, incensed by David's peremptory command, snapped, "Children do not talk to adults that way!"

All was lost. David winced, abandoned his plan, and tried to save the moment and regain some dignity by asking, "Why did you take blood from Katherine?" Shearer explained that he was looking for a marker that might indicate if she was a carrier of the defective gene. David made a remark about the new schedule, and it was all over. After Shearer left, David, humiliated, crumpled in my arms. "He didn't understand—no one understands—that I can't go on. What can I do to make people realize I can't go on? I wanted to talk, really talk."

David wept bitterly, I held him until the sobs subsided. I had to leave. I phoned Lynn several times. She said, "He's still huddled in a corner of the playroom yelling and crying, refusing all conversation."

That evening I tried—with little success—to console him, to explain how difficult it was for an adult to understand his maturity about this aspect of his life. Even if the conversation had gone according to David's script, I felt nothing would have changed.

David finally became more or less resigned to the new schedule. The remainder of his stay was spent with our playing hide-and-go-seek and long periods of silence. He lay on the floor of the playroom, and I lay on the windowsill near him. This was his way—or, I should say, our way—of grieving over our parting. "Mary, six months is eternity, two weeks a year is not enough of you."

"David, it's not just going to be two weeks a year. I'll visit you."

"Yes, it is. No matter what you say, it's just two weeks a year. Besides you, I have lots of friends here that I want to see—Potts, Jackie, Dorothy, and everybody, and there's Fannin Street."

"I know."

Dr. Desmond, Dr. Jay Tarnow, and I discussed my long silent periods with David. Dr. Desmond said, "This is too hard on you. It's too much for you to handle. Take two weeks vacation, go out of town, and when you return it will be over."

Jay and I, both stunned, said, "No."

"She could never leave him at this time," Jay explained. "She has to allow him to grieve and part."

Sunset had always been a special sharing moment for David and me. This summer the fiery, brilliant sunsets were more magnificent than ever. The evening before he left, David said, "The sunsets are always the same, yet each one is different; they're always beautiful, but this one is the most beautiful."

16.

AGE TEN—DAVID IS DISCHARGED FROM THE HOSPITAL

"Our being side by side reminds me of home when you stayed with me on Friday nights. You lay on the foam pad by the transport and we talked and talked and then slept all night. Now that I'm out of the bubble and in this room, we talk and doze and talk and doze all night."

"Difference was, at your house I slept good, happy to be with you." "Poor Mary. You haven't had a whole night's sleep since New Year's when my fever started."

"When you were sick and still in the bubble, yes, but since you've been out, I've been going home every other night."

"Yeah, I know you're alternating with my parents, but you're here early in the morning and late in the evening. So is Dr. Feigin, but he doesn't sleep in his office. Dr. Shearer does, and he calls me 'son.'"

"Things have changed between you and Dr. Shearer since the transplant."

"I never thought we would be friends. Remember the summer of '81 when he was not being understanding?"

"It's stamped indelibly on my mind: The new schedule of six months at home seemed like the end of the world. As it turned out, you were never at home for a full six months."

"Two times—almost."

"If you say so. What I remember is the disaster that Friday morning you left the hospital for the long stay at home."

"My mother was mad. You and Jackie looked sick. Jackie and I didn't expect you to refuse to get in the transport to go home. We were totally surprised."

That morning, July 31, 1981, Jackie and I sat with a resigned David waiting for Carol Ann, who arrived ninety minutes late. He saw her in the parking lot with his friend Shawn and stormed, "Why did she bring Shawn? I don't want him here!" He stood defiant in the far corner of the playroom and screamed to his mother, "I'm not going home! I want to talk in private." The loud discussion behind closed doors lasted over half an hour.

Finally, Carol Ann came out, and he was in the transport, ready to go.

For the first time, I experienced Carol Ann openly expressing anger.

"You should have warned me of David's state so I could have persuaded my husband to come!" she said. "Had he been here, there would have been no problem."

She did not listen when we insisted that we had not expected him to erupt. That afternoon, Lynn reported that when David was disconnected at home, he seemed calm and in good spirits.

David's going home the last day of July, not to return until December 11, entailed adjustment and ambivalence for all who loved him. As much as I would miss him, I couldn't help thinking, I have freedom. No more mad rushes during work hours, no juggling my social life or listening to "that boy comes first with you!"

For over a year the tensions and frustrations had run high among everyone involved with David. Many words, events, and reality itself contributed to the rift and anger between the family and medical staff, but thinking back, one decision taken by the doctors and one by the parents had inflamed the situation.

For the doctors' part, Drs. Shearer and Desmond, despite knowing David Sr.'s uncompromising opposition to "quack shrinks," had placed too much weight upon the psychiatric evaluation. No way could this practical, down-to-earth father accept an obscure psychiatric report as telling him anything meaningful about his son. On the other hand, the parents' blind faith in the expertise of the three original doctors was incomprehensible, especially since the three had long ago abandoned the sinking ship.

In retrospect, all of the bitterness would not have built up had Louise's advice of turning responsibility over to the parents been heeded, seven years before. At that time, David, at age three, was spending as much, if not more, time at the hospital than at home. Had the present schedule of six weeks home and two weeks at the hospital been in effect from that time on, more of the burden of the day-to-day behavior management would have fallen on the parents. The CRC staff and team would have been in the proper role of consultants, not "hospital parents." David would not have had to adjust to the diverse value systems of the hospital and the family.

But the rift had developed, and I was at the center of it. Three people with some degree of control over David's fate—Dr. Feigin, Carol Ann, and David Sr.—had no problem with my dual role as David's friend and a professional. Dr. Desmond and the assistant CDP indignantly voiced their belief that my personal involvement compromised my competence.

At Dr. Desmond's request, my work with David and the team was not included on the annual report of CDP's activities.

For some time I had been uneasy in the CDP meetings. It seemed as though my comments were unwelcome and resented, as if the underlying hostility of Drs. Shearer, Desmond, and Hansen was directed at me

Ultimately, my intuition of being the brunt of everything proved correct. During a team meeting, after a series of insensitive, belittling comments directed at me, followed by a disparaging remark from Dr. Shearer, Dr. Jay Tarnow sternly denounced them for using me as a "depository of feelings— feelings you can't admit to. You unconsciously see Mary in the role of a surrogate mother and as having taken on the responsibility for David's emotional life. She has become the depository for the feelings of the group. She is so involved and enmeshed with David that at times the boundary between the two is lost. She lives David's feelings very deeply and continuously represents him; therefore, this group projects their feelings onto her." No one commented.

One time Dr. Tarnow accused the team of using me as a "fire extinguisher." On another occasion he shocked them by referring to me as the "perfect mistress."

"You see, in reality, David's mother should have been his primary relationship," he told me. "Yet the two of you have such a powerful closeness that he has two women in his life. Like a mistress who seems to have a primary relationship with a man who is married, you are perfect because you don't ask for much nor let his mother know about the relationship you share with her son. I understand that you took on this role because of David's need for a protector during the hospital stays."

Dr. Tarnow was probably correct when he further stated that he sensed some tension between Carol Ann and me; however, he only observed us interacting in the tense group meetings. I don't believe David ever experienced any guilt over whom he should love, and Carol Ann's reliance upon me to take care of her son at the hospital prevented her from ever admitting, even to herself, any negative feelings toward me.

Nothing remarkable occurred the rest of the year. David reportedly adjusted well to the new schedule. Carol Ann's only concern was that he was not eating.

At David's tenth birthday in September, there would be no photos and no press conference—the first time these had been banned at his birthday. The September 1981 press release from Baylor read: "In consideration of David and his family, we did not take any pictures this year. During the past few years, David has shown some anxiety about having his picture taken and seeing himself in the newspapers and on TV. This concerns the medical staff, and they have asked us to wait awhile before taking more pictures. We will make every effort to have some new photos made as soon as possible."

The release included Carol Ann's statement: "One of the reasons we wanted David at home with us was to give him religious training, to share our faith with him. He is our son and this is where he belongs."

Carol Ann reportedly was encouraged with David's calm behavior on his birthday. He enjoyed the party with the extended family and took his First Communion.

In place of formal lessons, Carol Ann had been giving her son religious instruction. Miss Potts, Lynn, and The Methodist Hospital had struggled for six months to irradiate a wafer for Communion. The sterile wafer, which lost all of its texture, was consecrated after going in the bubble.

During my visits to his home, I found that the big item in David's life other than the *Star Wars* toys was a plastic cowboy hat, which he enjoyed wearing. He spent a lot of time with computer games and said, "You're no fun to play with—you don't get the hang of it." Renee, however, proved to be a challenging opponent.

When I visited on a Sunday afternoon in October, the fish, all dead, had been replaced by three parakeets, which flew around the room and perched on top of the bubble. I had visions of sharp claws piercing the PVC and parrot fever seeping through. Shawn, Katherine, and I struggled to catch the frightened birds and put them back in their beautiful cage.

I surmised, "No wonder your first parakeet expired so quick." The parakeets loose, together with Shawn and Katherine roughhousing and bumping into the bubble, made me a nervous wreck and I was relieved when Shawn left. David and I then had some private time and caught up on each other's news. He confided, "I'm making it and conforming, but it hasn't been easy."

Carol Ann was elated. "God has put Brynn Holcomb and Dr. Robert Good together." Both parents, eager to learn about Dr. Good's move to the University of Oklahoma, questioned me. All I knew was that he was leaving the Sloan-Kettering Cancer Institute. Carol Ann and David Sr. were confident that Dr. Good, "the father of immunology," who was to be provided with a modern, well-equipped lab and all the money he needed, would "come up with a cure for little David."

Not as enthralled as they, I merely said, "I certainly hope he does."

David returned to the hospital on December 11, 1981, for a one-week stay. Despite the obvious gaps in his experience, he was maturing: Avidly interested in current events, he could carry on an intelligent conversation on most any topic and all sports.

David had always noticed the clothes Jackie and I wore, but now he became quite critical of how we dressed. Jackie's dress, with a high neckline and very modest keyhole cut out, upset him no end; he considered it "indecent." He preferred for me to wear red, turquoise, and light blue. He "knew" I would not wear shorts or a sundress. On several occasions, he requested I stop by the hospital before going out to a social event so he could see me "all dressed up." On one occasion when I came by wearing a long dress, he said, "Oh my God, Mary! You can't go to a party in a nightgown with your hair in a wad on top!"

Jackie worried that TV distorted David's perception of the real world and family life. I made it clear to him that my lifestyle was atypical. Jackie confirmed that she, and indeed most people, did not own apartments in the Montrose area or have a world-traveling son. Her family, a husband and two daughters, was more the norm.

He understood this, but some of the simple things of life still went completely over his head. For example, on an episode of *The Jeffersons,* Mrs. Jefferson complained of having a bachelor houseguest outstay his welcome. What most annoyed her was his failing to put the toilet seat back down. David asked, "Why is a toilet seat so funny? How does it go up and down?" My explanations met with skepticism and, ultimately, "Forget it."

David's leaving for home on December 18 was uneventful. I promised to visit him during the Christmas holidays and did so on Wednesday, December 30. Once there, I reflected that I would not have traded places with Carol Ann in a million years. She had lost weight and looked strained, but was still ever so beautiful.

Aunt Patty had sent toys and pictures. David said, "Dr. Wilson's present must be delayed in the mail. I don't think he would forget."

From Carol Ann's comments, it was evident that she felt abandoned by the original three doctors.

David continued our routines at home, the same as in the hospital: hide-and-go-seek, clean birdcages (instead of fishbowls), gossip, and define words. I innocently thought we had been through all the risqué words: impotent, adultery, sterility, PMS, illegitimate, and brassiere. Now he came up with "What is birth control all about? I heard it on TV—there's no way anybody can control how many children they have. They just have 'em." He was fairly well versed in reproduction and knew that "doing it" did not always "make a baby."

"People can control how many children they have." "All right, explain it to me."

"The one sure way is to abstain from having sex. There are several other ways. The most popular one in use is the pill."

"The pill. I've heard of that but never understood what it was all about." "The woman takes a pill that stops the normal flow of the egg coming down each month, so conception never takes place."

"Okay, I got that, but you said several ways."

I went on to explain the diaphragm, condom, and the rhythm method.

"This is all a surprise. I never heard it before. Wait. Maybe I have. The pill and the rhythm have to do with the Pope. He's against a pill."

"Right. The Catholic Church forbids any artificial means of birth control. Using the rhythm method is permissible."

"That's nonsense. Either way, it's birth control." "Some other religions teach the same thing."

"Other religions? What other religions? There's only two—Catholics and Protesters. Why are you laughing?"

"My turn for surprise. I had no idea you thought there were only two religions. It's Protestant, not Protesters. Christian and Jewish are the main religious groups in this country."

"Jewish are a people, not a religion."

"It's both. Jews use the Old Testament and Christians use both the Old and New Testaments. You know the Bibles; we went through them long ago. Christianity includes Catholics and Protestants. Protestants have many subgroups—Lutheran, Episcopalian, and Baptist.... Other countries have other religions—Moslem in the Middle East, Buddhist in India, Shinto in Japan, and Confucians in China."

"This is news to me. Can you tell me about them all? Do you have books?"

"Yes to both."

For months we delved into the great religions of the world. He concluded the themes of each were basically the same.

I had an open invitation to visit David anytime. Whenever his mother took a weekend vacation, I stayed over on Friday night. During these quiet, enjoyable times, I came to know David's father well for the first time. A man of few words, he had a quick temper, which just as quickly subsided.

David, no doubt, acquired his creative building abilities from his father, a skilled cabinetmaker who made beautiful pieces of furniture. I don't think he shared this work with his son. One thing for certain, David's perception of a chair was totally different from that of his father. David's unorthodox, but correct, use of words and vocabulary are evident in his essay on a chair:

An object in this room is made up of wood and metal. It has four legs made of wood that are secured to the seat by a metal frame. The frame also supports a wood backrest. A chair in my room is made up of wood that is as tan as a Hawaiian's skin. The chair is also made of a metal frame. This frame is as silver as a nickel. The chair, in all, is as sturdy as an elephant's paw.

At the end of January, Bill phoned from the airport, "Mother, I have a surprise for you."

"Great. You've brought a Persian rug."

"No. I brought Lorna, the girl from the Philippines." Lorna, beautiful like the Polynesian girls in Gauguin's paintings, was like a breath of fresh air.

The summer before, when David had read Bill's letter from Abu Dhabi, he had exclaimed, "A girl! Bill's describing a girl! This is new! This must be serious. Do you think he will get married?"

"I don't know," I said. "It's the first real prospect." "Will he bring her here? I want to meet her. The Philippines—hmmm." I knew he would read the encyclopedia and question Kathy Jackson, his former teacher with whom he remained close.

Bill returned to the United Arab Emirates and left Lorna here for several months. Lorna knew of the famous Bubble Boy and could not believe she was going to meet him. David, frankly curious, wanted to meet the girl from Asia who had captured Bill's heart.

When Lorna and I arrived, David proceeded to amaze her with his knowledge—he pointed out that the Philippines are an archipelago of over seven thousand islands in the Pacific Ocean near China, the Mayan volcano erupts every ten years, and the dominant language is Tagalog.

He questioned her at length: "How did you meet Bill? Does Bill still have a beard? Would you like it if he shaved it off."

"I wouldn't mind at all," she replied in her halting English. "Bill can do whatever he wants. He looks pretty handsome with his beard."

"Handsome?" David said, mocking. "Bill, handsome? I don't remember what he looks like. I remember he's blond and tall, that's all."

"Well, at least you remember that he's blond and tall." David changed the subject, "Are you enjoying your stay in Houston?"

"A lot. A whole lot. I love the space of America—so spacious, so many things to buy, beautiful and accommodating people (she pointed to Carol Ann), and wonderful, nice, tall trees."

"It is interesting talking with someone from a foreign country who speaks a different language," David said. "I wish I could meet a person from every country in the world." Saying goodbye, he added, "It has been nice to meet you Lorna. Bill is lucky to have a pretty wife like you. Will you be coming back?"

She answered, "I'm not sure, but I'll try."

On the drive back, Lorna said, "He is such a good-looking young fellow—eyes so deep and meaningful. He's a very intelligent boy for his age. He talks like Bill, a man."

"Yes, he is very intelligent, but there are so many things he doesn't understand. He never forgets anything; he knows what Bill looks like."

On May 25, Jackie and I went to David's annual school show. He played the recorder and recited a poem by Shel Silverstein. The transport was disconnected and in the den. David, excited and nervous, had to urinate frequently, so every five minutes Jackie and I were holding up a sheet. Lynn and several nurses also attended. Other guests included the mothers of the children, Kathy Jackson, Carol Ann's close friends, several men from the Woodland's Golf Tournament, and Kent Demaret of *People* magazine.

Dennis Colburn, the school psychologist, after trying to counsel David, continued toward Carol Ann. David resented her talking to one of those "people I hate."

At the May 1982 CDP meeting, it was decided to repeat the psychiatric evaluation. My questioning the wisdom of this was interpreted as professional rivalry.

David, unbelievably furious when he learned that this hospital visit would be "spoiled" by an evaluation, confided, "I'll do or say something, and they will tell everybody I'm crazy. Then it will be that awful summer of '80 all over again. Mother will sit and stare, not talk, and Dad will be mad. I can't go through it again."

On the day David returned to the hospital, June 7, David Sr. restated to Dr. Shearer his firm position that his son would remain in the bubble until cured. Dr. Shearer described the latest work in immunology with unmatched bone marrow transplants.

The psychiatrist saw David for three one-hour sessions, and the psychologist saw him two days in a row. David admitted to rather liking the psychiatrist at times, but he resented his purpose: "to prove I'm crazy." The psychologist he simply "hated." Both men were impressed by David's memory of the previous evaluation, as well as his wit and sarcasm. They concluded that

David's state was very much as it had been two years ago, but he was now more depressed.

Tears, withdrawal, and constant complaints of "being tired" marked David's two-week stay. Jackie described a visit:

"David was very upset when I arrived. He had apparently lost two of his *Star Wars* figures, but his response was all out of proportion. He stayed extremely quiet, would not make eye contact, rocking and thumb sucking and some mumbling to himself. When I got ready to leave, he told me he was sorry he'd been so quiet, but that he was 'very tired.' I assured him it was okay and that I would see him on Monday at the regular time. His affect was the most depressed I have seen in the past year."

One evening, David, perspiring a lot, complained of being tired. Then, suddenly, an obviously sick pigeon landed on the window ledge. David almost went berserk, fearing that it would die then and there. There was absolutely no way for me to get to the bird; fortunately, it was soon dark. The next morning I rushed up, hoping against hope that the pigeon was not lying there dead. It was gone.

Not all our evenings were disasters. We followed the same old routines, hide-and-go-seek and roach patrol. David had a lot of catching up to do.

"Now that Bill has settled down, the only excitement left is Westheimer," he stated. The gay community in the Montrose area continued to be on the news, and he had many opportunities to see the "strange people" in the area.

David's favorite tenant was Wayne, who made pillows, decorated store windows, and cleaned apartments for me. Handsome Wayne dressed conservatively at times but also wore outlandish outfits—leather trousers and a vest with no shirt, and he sometimes wore one feather earring in an ear and the other earring in an exposed nipple.

David ordered, "Take a notepad with you every time you go there and jot down all the crazy outfits, count the couples—men holding hands and just plain girl-boy ones. I've figured out the Montrose area and Westheimer Street. It's a place my mother would never go."

"Right you are."

David continued an avid interest in current events and controversial issues. Between David and my mother, I never had to read a newspaper or watch the news; they kept me completely informed.

David's exit from the hospital to home on June 21 was swift and uneventful.

David called to discuss why all his parakeets died. (He had an endless supply from a family friend.)

"Other than your scaring them to death, I don't know." "No, I've been treating them better, but they still die.

"Those books you bought have no information. Buy another one, and get it in the cylinder Tuesday."

The book went off. He phoned.

"I got it figured out. It's the cage; the white paint contains lead. Please buy me another cage."

That weekend I took him a stainless steel cage. The parakeet lived for years.

David's new interest was child abuse. He knew of it from TV and the hospital. Now it was even closer to home; a six-year-old girl in Conroe had been raped and seriously injured. He knew the meaning of rape. Long ago, when he had heard of it on "All in the Family," I had defined rape as an act of violence against a person's body. His friend, Shawn, had filled in the details. His questions now went far deeper:

"Why would a grown man want to do it to a little girl? She wouldn't be sexually mature. You have to be fourteen to do it. Why?"

"You ask difficult questions, but I'll try. People develop and mature physically, mentally, and emotionally. You know all about mental retardation and such. We mature physically and sexually. Adults' hormones develop, and they have physical urges and take on an adult sexual partner. We also mature emotionally. When we're young, we select young playmates. As you grow older, you select people to interact with you who are at the same level of emotional maturity. Usually emotional and physical maturity go together, but not always. Probably what happened with the man who raped the girl is that he was physically and sexually mature, but not emotionally. Since his emotions were like those of a child, he would look for a child to relate to. Probably when he was with the girl, his physical urges took over. The little girl was there and he used her as a sexual object."

"Well, that makes sense. But it's still awful."

David's friend Shawn converted David's room at home into a TV repair shop. Although he was only a couple of years older than David, he was a whiz at electronics, and David enjoyed watching him work.

Shawn also provided David with an opportunity to indulge in some boys-versus-girl teasing, at my expense. In Shawn's presence, David asked, "Is this parakeet a male or a female?"

"I have no idea," I said.

He turned to Shawn saying, "See, I told you she wouldn't know—I told you she is dumb."

Shawn looked perplexed and said, "Her? Her dumb? No, not her. All that stuff she told you!" Not wanting to carry that subject any further, I remained silent.

I was more at ease and less anxious after David had a telephone. He could call when he wanted something and was now back into managing my business affairs.

When I visited in November, David's father and a nephew about David's age returned from deer hunting. The cousin came in holding a rifle and excitedly recounted stalking a deer. David, looking bewildered, couldn't follow the boy's narrative and finally asked to inspect the gun. I felt so sad and so helpless—David, not the cousin, should have been the one to go deer hunting with his father.

One day, David called to tell of watching *The Blue Lagoon* on cable TV. He related the story and expected me to fill in the "empty spots." I answered his questions about the ocean and living on an island, but not having seen the film, I was totally lost as to what happened from his description.

Later, I saw it and realized that he had done quite well in understanding the story. He had said, "The shipwrecked children and the ship's cook drifted onto an island. The man died, but they continued to follow his rule to not eat the berries. They did it, she got pregnant but they didn't know a baby was being born when she went into labor. They loved their baby a lot and played with it." He didn't understand the poisonous berries or the blood in the swimming scene (the girl's first menstrual period). "You've got two weeks before I come back to the hospital—that should give you time to find the answers." I called my friend, Barbara Miller, who taped the movie for me to view.

As surprising as it may seem, the questions David asked on sex and moral issues he got from the daytime soaps and the evening serials rather than the explicit cable TV movies. The soaps, apparently, cover all human frailties and sins. I cringed at some of the episodes on *Dallas* and *The Love Boat*. He did not need such exposure, but I could not dissuade him. As for the adult cable movies, he quit watching them because they were "all alike."

Mother and I attended David's eleventh birthday party. All the relatives from San Antonio were there; little cousins and other children ran around. At the last birthday party, David had been distressed when the kids absconded with his presents so now he demanded that they not touch them. His mother reprimanded, "It isn't polite."

This year he got in trouble by greeting guests with, "You cannot enter unless you have a present!" Carol Ann quickly put an end to that announcement.

David was pleased with my "IOU—One Present." He, in the disconnected transport and the vast table of food in the den, made for much tumult. My mother, totally overwhelmed, sat alongside him. She said, "I appreciate being invited, but it's too much."

David requested that the transport be moved out to the front yard. His father, several children, and I accompanied him. He had a ball, sprinkling with the hose. I had on a brand new red cotton skirt, and when it got wet, the red dripped on the bubble and everywhere. He yelled, "Get that red off!"

I once thought that if I ever wrote a book about David, it would be titled The Birthday Party. This party went well, but I recalled nightmarish ones. At age three, after the big hospital party with the VIPs and the news media, David had thrown a fit and told Dr. Wilson he never wanted another party. The problem was that he could not join in the celebration. At his four-year-old hospital party, he had held his hands over his ears and had refused to talk or visit with anyone. At one party, he'd had a cake that was shaped and decorated like a bubble.

Kay Miller vividly described the hospital birthday parties. "Oh, God, nobody wants to remember the damn birthday parties. Jesus, God, I don't. At one, David cried so hard we had to shut the doors. Horrible. You watch people who totally forget the child—everyone was in the limelight and David was forgotten. It was horrible. People were all around but he was alone—horrible."

David returned to the hospital on December 3, 1982, for a two-week stay. He now closely followed the controversy over the right to die—the legal, moral, and ethical issues of sustaining life on respirators, resuscitation after brain death, and tube feeding of comatose people.

His interest made sense. Having spent half of his life in a research center, he was familiar with terminal illness and degenerative diseases. Some children he had known who once walked around had become bedridden and vegetative. Also, he knew a great deal about leukemia. He could see children with no hair going in and out of the hematology clinic, a two-story annex by the parking lot, and he asked questions such as, "Why continue with medicine when there's no hope of ever being well?" He mulled over issues to which other ten-year-olds would never give a second thought. He identified with the terminally ill patients and realized his bubble was a life support system.

On December 5, David had a surprise birthday party for me, no guests. He gave me a silver letter opener. Nothing marred his visit this time. He enjoyed all his friends, and I visited every evening. He had grown so much, he was now fifty-five-and-one-quarter inches tall and weighed sixty-seven pounds, still slender. So ended 1982—the only year in which we did not spend a great deal of time together.

17.

ELEVEN—THE AGE OF REASON

"All of 1983 was different. So much happened. One good thing, we had lots of time together. Right, Mary?"

"Right. You phoned on January 14 to tell me you were coming back for a few days while the playroom blower system was being repaired. Jackie and I met you. Happy three days. Even the flood didn't faze you."

"At four-thirty in the morning the water main over the playroom burst. Lynn came in, put the motors up, capped off the transport and crib, and turned the playroom blowers off because the electrical plug was in water. Mr. Langford had to come in early!"

Lynn, now head nurse, had trained a nurse's aide, Delores Johnson, to carry out the mundane duties of keeping the isolator system going. Eleven-year-old David, always miles ahead of Delores, wasn't bothered by her constant nagging. She was a source of information—she attended the CDP meetings and he elicited every scrap of information from her without her ever realizing it.

Each time Delores went to the house, the bubbles were a mess. What she didn't see he told her on the phone and kept her in a perpetual snit. For example, her log note: "David stated he had spilled urine in the playroom. David was instructed to get all of the urine up. [The next day] David stated that he 'hadn't gotten the urine up' and also he had three days of trash inside the isolator. I stated to David that it had been two days since he spilled... I told

David about how the trash would grow bacteria, and if he fell and slipped and cut his finger... We would have to bring him back to the hospital." Lynn had to step in and chastise both David and Carol Ann. The problem of punctures, splits, and pulled away sleeves kept Delores busy.

On my home visit, David was in a smart-aleck mood, and after his grandmother and mother went shopping, he ordered, "Get a trash bag. We are going to clean house." I sorted through piled high shelves and a large box full of junk as he directed whether to trash or to save. "All of Dr. Wilson's cards go in the trash."

"Think about that, David; he's your godfather," I cautioned.

I got a dirty glare and an emphatic "In the trash!" When his mother and grandmother returned, he nastily said, "Look, Mary had to do all your work!"

I reprimanded, "If either one touched your stuff, you would have thrown a fit."

"Yeah," he agreed.

I had long wanted to write a paper on David's unique perceptual development. Carol Ann not only gave me permission but also encouraged me to write it. Next, I discussed it with David.

"It's all right with me," he said. "You're wasting your time. I don't think anyone will be interested, but I bet they would be interested in a paper about our private world. Do you think anyone could understand a relationship between a boy and an older woman? I know, we should write a book and the title will be 'The Boy in the Isolator and the Woman Who Never Touched Him.'"

"You're probably right. Tell you what—you start on the book and I'll start on the paper."

"Maybe I will. What help do you need from me on the paper? Will it be like your other papers with all the literature first?"

"Yes."

Several weeks later, David phoned, "You must be here by six-thirty on Friday night. There's a movie on cable you have to see."

"If it's another *Halloween II*, forget it."

"Oh, now it wasn't that bad. I told you when to close your eyes. This is different. It's beautiful, no blood and you'll like the music. I checked with Mother. It's fine for you to come."

On Friday evening, David told me, "I know you're not interested in and don't understand space science fiction, but *Star Trek* is different. You don't have to understand anything about the spaceship. The end is what is important."

This was the first of the *Star Trek* movies. The story centered on the need of VGER (the space ship Voyager on a 300-year journey of data collection for NASA) to evolve beyond pure logic into the realm of human emotion. In merging with two living creatures, Captain Decker of the starship *Enterprise* and the Delton girl, VGER will survive by becoming one with its creator. In dazzling beauty and to exquisite music—the luminous sparks from VGER becoming yellow and purple spheres swirling around all three—they drift off, evolving into a new, higher life form that has the ability to create its own sense of purpose.

"See—that is the way it is in eternity. We simply evolve into a higher life form, touch God and find answers," David said decisively. "It is exactly like Bill's *Eternity*. It's like you've always said, 'There is life and there is death; they are both part of the same process—death must be beautiful.'"

The next Sunday morning, I phoned David and got no answer. I didn't think too much of it. They could have been putting in supplies, or maybe they had taken him outside for a while—unusual, but possible. At four o'clock, still no answer. This was unusual. David was many things, but hard to find was generally not one of them. I called CRC—they knew nothing. I couldn't stop worrying. As I was leaving to drive to Conroe, the phone rang.

"Mary!" said David, sobbing. "Love, what's wrong."

"Oh, Mary, that was you calling all afternoon wasn't it? I knew it was you—I could feel it."

"Yes, I was just going out the door to come see what was going on." "My phone's broke and they forgot to set the kitchen one in here. I could hear it ring, but there was nothing I could do. I knew it was you and I knew you'd be upset."

"What's wrong with your phone?"

"I'm not sure, but I think it's that little thing that plugs in. Why?"

"I'll buy all the things it takes to fix it and bring them up. Not tonight, but next weekend."

"Maybe you should check with Mr. Langford. He knows all about these things."

On Friday evening I replaced the cord. He grinned and said, "Thanks Miss Fix-It. We can't make it without a phone, can we?"

On May 27, 1983, Delores, Marla Wolf, R.N., and Irene Wattington, R.N., transported David to the hospital, and Lynn followed in a car. Lynn, who was to leave the first of August, had trained these two. The first evening back and every evening of the stay, our conversations centered on David's feelings of despair and on suicide:

"Suicide is terrible. Don't you agree—suicide is an awful thing?" "That's a bit difficult to answer yes or no. The Catholic Church is very much against suicide. It used to be that if a person committed suicide they couldn't be buried with all the sacraments and in a church cemetery. But, the more important thing is to first define suicide. Many people consider any intent to terminate life as suicide. I don't. If someone has something go wrong in their life and they jump off a roof or shoot themselves, that's suicide and I agree it's terrible. It's wrong. But I also believe if someone has a terminal illness, it's their right to stop treatment that prolongs life and suffering to no avail. People should be allowed to die in comfort with dignity."

"What you mean is, if they're in the hospital, and they're suffering, they might just want the peace of going home, and that would be all right. It wouldn't be suicide to stop the medicine?"

"That's what I believe," I said.

"Well, you know what I think? I think suicide is a personal decision." "It's not always simple. A person may be too ill or too young to use good judgment. They need help in making a decision. Possibly their situation is not as hopeless as they believe."

"What about comatose people on life support systems?" "It can be a dire dilemma. It's the same as the medication. Although the Catholic Church is very specific in stating that suicide is a sin, it does not believe in sustaining life just to prevent death. Death is natural. A Hindu near death does not want to be in a noisy intensive care unit because he believes the way you enter the next world has very much to do with the state you are in when you leave this world. Ideally, each hospital should have a team—the clergy, a physician, a layperson, and an ethicist to assist families in making a logical decision in a time of stress.

"That's what they should have for some of those tiny preemies they put on respirators and never take off."

David was intent on our watching the movie *Murder For Love*, for which he had seen previews. The story involves two brothers: one of them, a young man who lies paralyzed and in pain, pleads with his brother to kill him to end his misery. Because the brother loves the injured man, he shoots him. At the end of the movie David inquired, "Would you do that for me? You don't have to answer. Anyway, you couldn't shoot anybody for any reason."

"You're right, I won't even touch a gun."

"Mary, let's play hide-and-go-seek and talk about this later. It's too depressing."

While we had our share of morbid conversations, many more were mixed—David would alternately reassure me that he was fine and complain that life was awful. For example, one evening David asked, "How do you feel about me being in this bubble? I know you feel sorry for me being in here."

"That's not exactly right. I don't feel sorry for you, I feel sad that you must live in there."

"I don't know why. I'm happy in here. We have good times, and we're good friends, so why should you be sad?"

"I want you to experience and do the things my son did."

"But we do lots of things together. We're friends. What else do we need?"

"We could hold hands and walk around, sit under a tree, look at the whole sky, see all the stars, and jump in water."

"I don't want to stay home so long. You don't understand, two weeks a year isn't enough time with you."

"I see you more than two weeks a year."

"It's just two weeks. No one cares anything about me anymore. Nobody cares what happens to me. Everybody's lost interest. And let's face it; I've lost interest in everything. I wish Dr. Shearer had been more understanding when I tried to talk to him about what would happen if I came out. Those three doctors that put me in here left because they didn't know what the hell to do with me. I'm losing interest in everything at home and my family, and the truth of the matter is they are tired of me. How much does it cost to keep me in here?"

"We've been through your compulsive doubting before. You're wrong about your family losing interest. It's just that your living at home for such a long period is a strain on everybody, especially your mother."

"You're right. She's just as trapped as I am. The house is her bubble."

David changed the subject. "I've given a lot of thought to the stock market. I think we could do just as good with a random selection. If I make a selection will you buy the stock?"

"Okay. How are you planning to do this?"

"Open up the paper *(The Wall Street Journal)* to the stock market, and I'll take a pencil, close my eyes, and jab."

"You can jab, but if it's over fifty dollars a share, you'll have to jab again." "Fine, get off the New York Exchange page." He jabbed Quadrex. I bought a hundred shares at six dollars a share.

Martha Currie, the new CRC head nurse, followed the van to David's home on June 10, so his departure went smoothly. At the June 13 CDP meeting, Jackie and I said little, as we knew he would learn everything that we said from Delores. Afterward, Jackie reflected, "How many meetings have we sat through and listened to everybody talk when you and I were the only ones who knew what was going on in that room upstairs?"

I wrote a letter to Drs. Desmond and Shearer summarizing David's despair and quoting his comments on suicide.

One weekend at Conroe, David was helping to plan my trip to Singapore.

"It certainly is far away. Look at the globe. It's halfway around the earth." "I want to tour the Orient with Bill, but I dread the twenty-eight hours of flying to get there."

"Well, if you don't like flying that long, why don't you just drive?"

His father joined us laughing and shaking his head, "There are some things my son just doesn't get."

"I can't drive to Singapore." "Sure you can."

"It takes a week to drive to California—then there's the Pacific. What would I do?"

"Drive across it."

"I'd sink. You can't drive on the ocean." "Take a ship."

"It takes two weeks to sail across the ocean."

"No, six weeks of travel is too long. Let's figure this one out with the globe. I think you could drive the other way."

The exchange went on and on. I had thought he had a better understanding of time and distance. Obviously, the magnitude of the trip mystified him and the vast expanse of the Pacific Ocean eluded him.

He threw his hands up. "You should probably just go ahead and fly."

David phoned. A Houston Oiler football player, Earl Campbell, had visited. The player's size impressed him. "You wouldn't believe how big he is—his legs, wow—one thigh is bigger than me, or even you, and his skin is really black."

"Was he interesting to talk to?"

"No. We exchanged words, and I asked questions. He's coming back again."

On Sunday, David called, disappointed. "He hasn't shown up. He called Friday and said he would be here Sunday afternoon."

"Maybe you misunderstood the day."

"No. Why would he say one thing and then do another? Don't bother to answer—he's like most people—you can't believe 'em."

A barrage of questions followed. After an hour, I suggested we get off the phone; the football player might be trying to call. He lambasted, "You're like everyone else, you're tired of me."

"No, that's not it. We shouldn't stay on the phone so long. Let's make more calls and have shorter conversations."

"Can I call you back later?" "Certainly."

He called Monday evening—the same nothing. Tuesday evening he told of his gossip session with Delores.

"I needed to stir up some excitement. I told her I knew all about sex." Shawn was a secret source of information.

"I bet her voice screeched straight up."

That week David called every night and asked the same trivial questions. Finally, he admitted having a problem. "I need to talk. Can you come visit this weekend? I'll get permission."

In a few minutes, Carol Ann called to invite me to a buffet dinner and poker party the coming Friday. "You're welcome to visit with David, or we would be happy if you'd play poker."

The bizarre Friday evening started with a great dinner, shrimp and eggplant soufflé and other gourmet dishes. I knew I was in for a profound conversation with David—it had been coming for several months. I feared he had made a decision and had immediate intentions to carry it out.

As soon as we finished dinner, he ordered me to take a bath while he saw to my bed being fixed. "We can whisper if I lay in the transport and you lay with your head right next to mine," he said.

The noise from the blowers and the party in the next room would make it difficult to hear whispers, I complained.

"Go buy a hearing aid because I have lots of questions. Why doesn't my mother care about me anymore?"

"I don't think that's true."

"Yes, it is. It's true. She doesn't care about me or how I feel. Believe me, I know she doesn't care."

"Well, I know she does care."

"But sometimes she doesn't talk and won't look at me and doesn't listen. Sometimes she just sits and stares."

"When people care so much about someone, and something isn't right, it hurts too much. So much that they can't stand to think about it. The pain is too great; they deny the problem exists. They do it because if they face it, they hurt too much."

"Do you think that's what she's doing?"

"Yes. I know she cares very much. I think there are times when she has to withdraw from everything. Also, she's very tired."

"You're right. I know my parents love me. But love isn't enough. I can't—no one can—make it on just love. Oh, Mary, look at you—look at us—proof. Long ago love was enough, but not now and not tomorrow. You're worried about me and the teenage years. I know exactly how you feel about me being in here, but you're wrong—I am happy. What can I do to convince you that I'm happy in this bubble? I don't want to come out. I love my bubble, and I love being in here."

"You're right. You could never convince me."

"Why?"

"Oh, David, come off of it. You've called me every night for more than a week, teary and complaining about 'poor little me.' Just now, you told me you're convinced that no one cares. How can you expect me to believe you when you say you're happy?"

"Yeah. But tell me why you're unhappy about me." "You know I feel what you feel."

"I know that, but why else?"

"Because you can't do all the things you could do if you were out. Whenever you say you're happy, my own feelings interfere. So, you could never convince me."

"So I won't try. What does Dr. Shearer feel about me?" "As a physician and a scientist, he is frustrated."

"Okay, okay. Now I've got one more to ask and I want you to promise you'll answer. You might think this question is foolish, but will you promise to answer? Maybe you won't want to answer my question. Maybe you can't answer. Do you think I should come out?"

"You posed the question in such a way as to expect a yes or no answer," I said carefully. "It's difficult to answer yes or no. One part of me says yes, come out, and we'll run outside and do the things we've talked about. A part of me says, 'do that'—take your chances, do things and have fun—even if for a short time. Then, another part of me says no, don't come out. We don't know how long you'll have or what will happen. I can't bear the thought of not having you. My little friend, you are a part of me. My love, I wish most of all that you could come out cured."

"I knew what you'd say. You would never make that decision for me. But no matter what, you'll be with me."

"I need time."

"Yes. I'll tell you what let's do—go to sleep." Believe it or not, despite the enormity and far-reaching implications of our dialogue, we both went to sleep immediately.

Before leaving the next morning, I again encouraged David to talk with his father.

"You know we don't talk, we merely exchange words."

"Listen to me. You're a master at controlling conversations and too quick to cut people off. Give your father a chance; you two can talk."

"No, I can't. I couldn't bear to see the pain in his eyes if I tell him. He wouldn't understand that love is not enough. Neither would my mother."

"Maybe. But please try." "No. It's you and me."

Driving home I felt relieved. Although David was moving toward a decision, he wasn't planning a rash move. I had time. He knew I would talk with Dr. Feigin after I thought things through. Finally, on Thursday, August 11, 1983, I had my three-page note written. I summarized my conversation with David. I asserted my belief that David had every right to make a decision because he had reached the age of reason.

Then everything changed.

That Thursday evening, David phoned. "How are you?" His voice cracked. "I'll see you in a few days. I'm coming into the hospital for a monoclonic transplant."

I nearly dropped the phone. "David, what did you say?"

"I'm coming in for a monoclonic transplant—they clone out the T-cells of the donor so I won't get graph-versus-host disease. My father decided."

"When?"

"I don't know, a few days ago. Maybe yesterday, maybe a week," said David, sobbing softly. "Will you come out tomorrow night and talk?"

"Yes."

"Okay. See ya."

One minute later, Carol Ann called. "My husband and I talked to Dr. Shearer last Friday. Of the two methods for an unmatched bone marrow transplant, he advises the monoclonic antibody. Tuesday my husband phoned him. We decided to go ahead with a monoclonic transplant. Little David is very upset," she continued. "We asked him if he wanted to talk to you, but he said he wanted time first. Would you please come out and convince him it's okay? I really want you to talk to him—it might ease his mind. We have a film that explains the procedure. I'm going to be away for the weekend, but my husband will be here."

First thing the next morning, I made an appointment to see Dr. Feigin, but it was half past three before he was available.

"I'm annoyed at learning of the transplant from David himself," I told him. "Why didn't you tell me? His parents want me to persuade him. How am I supposed to go up there and convince him to go through a procedure I know nothing about?"

"The parents initiated the request," Dr. Feigin said. "I think it's worth the risk. Probably the worst that can happen is that nothing will happen."

"I planned to give you this note today." I handed it to him, and he read it silently. Although the note made it clear that I felt David should make the decision, he inferred from it that he and the parents were on the right course.

"Yes, it's the thing to do," he said.

"You know there is one thing David will want." "Mary, you'll be there."

"How is it done?"

"You'll have to ask Bill, but it's not complicated or painful." I phoned David from Dr. Feigin's office to tell him that I was on my way. I drove for over two hours through torrential rain. David was beside himself and in tears, certain I'd had an accident.

He was clearly happy to see me, but quickly started flipping videotapes from one box to another. "Oh, Mary, I'm in one of my frantic moods."

"Okay, David, let's see the video."

It was a news broadcast, taped by a friend, describing the successful monoclinic antibody treated transplant of a little girl at Boston Children's Hospital. Old film clips showed David in the bubble and the space suit. The commentator stated that David, the most famous immune deficient child in the world, had no need for a transplant because the space suit allowed all the mobility he needed.

David started crying.

"Did you hear that? He said 'mobility.' Mobility? On that lousy day? You know! You were there! You're always there when it's a lousy day and that was really a lousy day. Every time I've ever had a lousy day you've been with me. If they do this thing, that will be a lousy day, so will you be there, too? You will be there?"

"Yes."

"How do you know?" "Dr. Feigin assured me."

"Oh, damn, why did you talk to Dr. Feigin?"

"Listen, you phone and tell me you're going to have a monoclonic transplant. I can't even pronounce the name, let alone spell it. I should come up here and talk when I know nothing? I needed answers. He is the only one I can talk freely with."

"Oh, all right, Miss Reality. How can I trust that procedure when that film is so wrong about me? You heard it. They said 'mobility.' "

"That newscaster didn't know. He just put the story together from the NASA films. But doctors have perfected the cloning technique."

Just then David Sr. came home and joined us. He was pleased that I had talked with Dr. Feigin. "That's really great that you can be with him during the procedure. What is Dr. Feigin's opinion?"

"He thinks it's worth the risk."

David Sr. went out to buy hamburgers, and a furious David let me have it. "You didn't have to agree with him! Why couldn't you keep your blankety-blank mouth shut? I know what you said in the kitchen! You'd do anything to get me out of here! Mary Ada, I knew you'd agree to the transplant, but did you have to agree so quick?"

"In the kitchen," I said, "we discussed what kind of hamburger I wanted. I have not agreed to anything. I'm up here to talk—not to make a decision that is not mine to make."

"Oh. All right. Tell me everything Dr. Feigin said."

"It's a simple procedure, not painful, and he thinks it is worth the risk. There is risk."

"I have no choice in the matter and, what's more, I decided I don't want it. There's nothing I can do. Oh! There might be something I can do! What if I call the news people and tell them I've no choice, and I don't want a transplant. I bet they'd be interested—they'd listen!"

"Enough! Enough!"

He paused and calmed a little, and so did I.

"I figured it out," he said. "Three things bother me. Number one, I'm afraid of the procedure—the transplant itself. Number two, I'm afraid I'll get my hopes up, and then it won't work. And number three, I'm afraid that it might work, and I won't be able to adjust to coming out."

"Let's take them one at a time. Number one is not going to be a problem. I'll be there."

"Dr. Feigin's word is law. So you'll be there."

"Yes. As for number two, we've talked before about risk. Without risk, you gain nothing. Most anything worthwhile in life requires some risk. If we decide to love or be a friend, we risk being hurt in that relationship. We risk hurt many ways with money, time, and effort. But if we never took a risk, life would be dull—no pleasure, no possessions, no achievements. If human beings never took risks, we'd still be sitting in a cave."

"Yeah."

"As for number three, I don't think coming out will be easy, but we can take it one step at a time. It can be done gradually, and I'll be with you each step. So will Jackie."

"I know you'll do that, but it's too late. I could have handled coming out better several years ago."

"Probably so. I think you could talk to your father about this." "Oh, come on."

We talked for over two solid hours. Over and over he stated the three fears, and I came back with all the answers I knew. I was determined that he was going to talk to his father in the morning. We played hide-and-go-seek for a while and then went to sleep.

The next morning, the three of us viewed the film together. I pointed out that the newsman, not the doctors, had used the term "mobility." I mentioned David's three fears. His father said, "I know it's very frightening." He seemed quite sensitive and understanding about his son's concerns.

David Sr. prepared breakfast for me, and we conversed briefly. He thanked me for coming up and talking with David. "After all, you, too, are his mother," he said. "He trusts you, and he trusts us, and I think this is the thing to do."

I asked, "Why did you come to this decision?"

"Several friends and clients showed me a newspaper article on this treatment, and one made the video tape. I think it's time to do something."

"I agree. The last time I was here, David wanted to talk about the future—the reality of being an adult in a bubble. I have seen similar realizations in cerebral palsy children. They know when they are little that they'll be CP when they're grown up, but it is only at about age twelve that the realization of what it actually means to be an adult CP sets in. Then you have a period of depression. David's in that depressed stage."

"He talked to you about that?"

"Not exactly in those words. But he has reached the point where he believes being a teenager or an adult in the bubble is intolerable."

"I appreciate all the time you spend with David, especially last night, and I'm glad you talked with Dr. Feigin." He hit his fist on the table. "We're going to do it!"

18.

A COCKROACH AND EXPLODING TURTLES

"Mary, when this is all over, who will take care of you?" He didn't expect an answer and went on, "Remember last August when Hurricane Alicia knocked out the power? I couldn't breathe and the bubbles fogged up. I had to come back to the hospital."

"David, I'll never forget that Thursday morning when the eye hit. The sky was green and the wind stopped. You were frantic on the phone."

On August 18, 1983, I called David about half past ten in the morning after the hurricane passed.

Carol Ann answered. "We were just trying to call you. David is tense and wants to talk to you. Our power is out. You must have had a good talk with him when you were here last weekend."

"Yes."

"I thought so, because he seems to accept the idea of the transplant better now. He's anxious to talk... hold on."

"I'm in one of my frantic moods. I was so worried about you. The eye of the hurricane went through right where you live. Now it's on its way to Conroe and the generator won't work."

"Settle down... tell me just exactly what is happening."

"I've only got forty-five minutes of air left. Don't make me explain how I know."

"Surely the fire department will come with one." "They already did. They need a bigger one."

"Just calm down. Everything is going to be all right. I promise. I'll call back in thirty minutes."

When I called back he didn't have time to talk. A big truck with a big generator was there and he had to "supervise."

On August 20, Marla and Delores went out to the house and brought David back to the hospital. I was grateful to go to work that day—I had no electricity and it was hot and humid. David decided, "Spend all your time at the hospital with me. Don't go to a hot house: Let's not mention you-know-what—they eavesdrop and write it in my chart."

David busied himself checking on the minor hurricane damages on my various properties, such as the lightning that had struck the garage apartment on Westheimer.

Saturday evening, I chalked up feeling lousy, tired, and having a headache and a stiff neck to sleeping with no air conditioning and running myself ragged. Sunday evening, while with David, I realized the excruciating pain was a toothache.

I called my dentist, who prescribed immediate antibiotics and told me to be at his office at seven in the morning.

"Be sure to drink your coffee here before you go," David ordered. The next morning he instructed, "Carefully watch everything so you can tell me about it. And while you're there, ask him about that black line on your tooth. I don't like it. They will be taking pictures, and it might show. Be sure to come back up here just as soon as you get back."

When I returned from the dentist, David declared, "Oh! Oh! Mary Ada, you look awful! You might faint. Sit down. What happened? What did he say to do?"

"He pulled my tooth. He said go to bed and put ice on my face."

"Now, Mary, you leave everything to me. I'm taking charge." He ordered the nurse to bring a bag of ice, a pillow, and a chair. He told me, "Sit in your little chair, but first put it right next to the transport so I can touch you. Put the pillow on the big chair, then put the ice on the pillow, and put your cheek on it. I'll call Mildred and tell her where you are."

I lucked out; my eight-thirty appointment was a no-show. I immediately went to sleep. David gently woke me saying, "Your ten-thirty kid is here. As soon as you're finished testing, you come back. It's best if you stay here with me so I can take care of you. Don't go home to no air conditioning. Don't go back to your office and be alone."

Wednesday, August 24, the utilities were back on at David's house and he went home. Carol Ann followed the van. Somehow, Marla and Delores went on Highway 59 instead of Highway 45, losing their escort. Halfway home, David complained of nausea and not being able to breathe. Wet with perspiration, he vomited. Everyone was relieved when the trip was over.

Over a month had gone by since David's parents had asked for the transplant, and no date for the operation was set. The tissue analysis and arrangements took time. David and I, mistakenly, had expected it to be over by now. Each day everyone's anxiety accelerated, and David worried, "What if it's in October and you're in Singapore?"

"I've postponed the trip."

"No, don't do that—let's postpone the transplant."

"Too late, I've canceled my reservation. I had call forward pushed on my phone so you can keep up with me."

David invited me to his twelfth birthday party on Wednesday, September 21, 1983. No guests—only his parents, Katherine, and me. Although he was pleased at having a "private" party, Carol Ann felt guilty about not having the energy to prepare the usual big event. The truth was that none of us was up to being with a lot of people. No photographs were taken for a news release.

A week before his birthday, David decided to have the party on the Friday before his birthday so I could stay all night. When I phoned from home, Carol Ann said, "I am grateful you are spending Friday night with us. I need to talk. All I can do is sit, and look at the wall."

"Carol Ann, call Dr. Hansen," I said. Despite the concern David Sr. had about "quack" psychiatrists, this struck me as a situation so stressful that a professional was needed.

But she refused. "No. We haven't told the children yet that Katherine will be the donor. I'm so afraid the transplant won't work."

She again adamantly opposed seeing Dr. Hansen. I finally said, "If you won't call him, can you hold on until I get there tomorrow? I'll leave early "

Carol Ann had every reason to be stressed out. I was concerned about her, but also about how her emotional state would affect David. My anxiety level high, I didn't know how to help her.

So, I went to ever-supportive Barry Molish. "I need an hour of your professional time. I'm on the verge of collapse." I briefly told him of the impending transplant and Carol Ann's state.

"I don't think it's the transplant itself," he said. "It's something else. Most likely she wants to be the donor. She feels since she passed along the defective gene that might rectify things. Now, instead, both of her children are placed in jeopardy. She wonders if she is being fair to each." He paused and looked me squarely in the eye. "I'm going to lay out a dialogue to follow." For the next hour, he did exactly that, anticipating Carol Ann's questions and giving me appropriate responses.

I managed to leave early for Conroe. The hour's drive, during which I rehearsed Barry's script, allowed me to step back and gain some composure and confidence.

Walking in the unlocked front door, I immediately confronted two portraits of pain: David rocking on his knees in the transport and Carol Ann sitting on the den couch. Neither seemed to hear me call out, "I'm here." For the first and only time in almost ten years, I saw Carol Ann without makeup— nothing could have been a clearer sign that something was terribly wrong.

My God, I thought. Which one do I go to first? David, of course.

He looked like a zombie. In place of the usual spontaneous greeting, he spoke in an eerie, slow cadence: "M-a-r-y, i-t i-s s-o n-i-c-e o-f y-o-u t-o c-o-m-e." The transplant being the only thing on my mind, I assumed his catatonic stupor was due to his tension about it and Carol Ann's state. Things were far worse than I had imagined.

"David, look at me—look!" I said. After a long silence tears came. "A roach got into my playroom."

Caught totally off guard, I staggered visibly—it hadn't occurred to me that something else had happened. When I found my voice, I asked, "When did you find the roach?"

"I didn't. It was in the hospital playroom."

Completely stunned for a second, I was suddenly overcome with rage.

"Who told you?"

"You're upset. I can tell. I can tell by your eyes. You're upset. You're really upset. You can't stand straight. You're just as upset about the roach as I am."

"I'm not as upset about the roach as I am about the fact that they told you, not me. Where is it now?"

"It's dead and out. Did you want them to lie to me?"

"No, but I should have been told first. How did you find out?"

He refused to say.

"If anything would have ever gotten in the bubble, we should have known it would be a roach," I said, trying to put it in perspective. "They've survived since the beginning of Earth. They are everywhere."

As he continued to lament over the roach, I was struck by the impossibility of the situation. As if the transplant were not enough—now, a damned roach!

Carol Ann went to the grocery store. For an hour, David and I discussed all the possible ways the roach might have entered the isolator. His belief that it came through the filter system was probably correct.

"Roaches can burrow through the media filter but a germ would get stuck," I said. I added that it would be simple to prevent in the future—just tape a screen over the intake.

Today appeared to be the day for troubles from the animal kingdom. I heard a weak cry from under the bubble, and David said, "That's a kitten Katherine found. You have to feed it every twenty minutes while you're here." I'm usually sympathetic to waif animals, but at the time, I was not interested in nursing a newborn, flea infested kitten that appeared to be on its last legs.

David then informed me the parakeet needed attention. It looked like hell, color faded and neck swollen. I asked him when he had fed it last. He didn't remember. The birdseed box was empty. "As soon as somebody comes back, they're going out to get food for this wretched bird. Where is your father?"

"He's at the lake exploding turtles." "He's what?"

"Exploding turtles. That's what he said." Weirdness upon weirdness.

When Carol Ann returned, I told David she and I were going to talk. He doubled over, moaning. "You can't talk to her! I don't want you to talk to her! You might say the wrong thing! I don't want you to talk about me!"

"I am going to talk to her. She and I need to talk. You won't be the topic of conversation. Stop whimpering. You've got your TV program coming up—watch it while we talk."

Barry's script went smoothly. He had predicted accurately Carol Ann's every statement: Both my children are in danger. Am I being fair to David? Am I being fair to Katherine? I want to be the donor. It would be only right for me to be the donor. Using Barry's words, I encouraged her to talk, realizing that there were no answers to most of these questions, but that it would help her to vent her feelings. The talk was good for both of us. After a while she moved to another subject:

"I have come to appreciate Dr. Shearer and his attitude. At first I resented the fact that no personal relationship existed, but now I'm glad it doesn't. I haven't discussed the transplant with Dr. Wilson and I don't want to."

"I think that's wise," I said. "Why?"

"He's so far removed from what's going on. Also, you once told me that he could persuade you to do anything, and he implied the same to me."

"Looking back, I'm angry with him," she said. "I wasn't persuaded because of his knowledge but because of religion. He stood for my religion and for what was right."

"I don't think you could have separated the two." Katherine came breezing in. David told her we were celebrating his birthday early. She was now a strikingly pretty girl of fifteen. I had never seen her hostile before, but apparently the tension was getting to her, too.

"Next Wednesday is not a birthday, it's a curse day! The day you were born was the beginning of a curse on this family!" she shouted. As she continued with this tirade, David took it for a while but then began screaming back at her. Carol Ann walked in at that moment and immediately chastised him.

I am not a drinking person, but if I were, by then I would have been dead drunk. Instead, I went on a chocolate binge. I devoured a bowl of chocolates by going back in the den for one more, one more, one more, until they were gone. David cautioned, "Mary, you'll get sick."

At that moment, David's father walked in holding a big rifle. "Explain exploding turtles," David requested.

"The turtles are eating all the fish in a lake that belongs to a friend of mine, so I shoot them. When they're hit, they explode."

David shook his head. "It's just the tension from living." After dinner, David and I again discussed his three worries and his desire to say no to the transplant.

"You said no to the space suit and that was the end of it. If you said no to the transplant, Dr. Feigin would listen to you," David insisted.

"This is different from the space suit. I do not have the right to say yes or no, and you really don't want me to say no to a transplant."

"You're right. If just it would be over with, and I could quit being afraid of the procedure itself."

"I've told you to put that worry to rest. I'll be there, and everything will go fine."

David brought up the current press release, which told of his going to a theater for a private viewing of *Return of the Jedi*.

"Why are people so interested?" He asked. "I just don't understand. I wonder why my mother has never talked to a reporter."

"She did when you were little."

"I bet they'd be interested in the transplant and really interested if they knew I was saying no. Tell you what, let's play hide-and-go-seek."

The next day, when I left, everything was calm. David seemed at ease, and Carol Ann was herself again, composed and beautiful.

On the drive back, I fantasized gruesome things to do to the CRC staff for needlessly terrifying David. In the end, I never ever mentioned the roach to them. Instead, I wrote Dr. Shearer a scathing letter saying, in essence, that if Donna or Lynn were still here instead of the present stupid staff, the incident would never have happened. Later I learned that everyone on CRC staff knew I was madder than hell.

A wonderful thing happened during this awful period. "Mother," said Bill on the telephone, "come April you'll be a grandmother! Any names in mind?"

David, exuberant, never viewed the baby as a rival. But he also urged me to fill Bill in on the transplant before it was revealed in the press. (As yet, only the family, Drs. Feigin and Shearer, the Boston people, and I knew about the transplant.)

When I told him, I was unprepared for Bill's violent opposition.

"Stop it!" he demanded. "Mother, you can't go along with an experiment to kill Little Brother!"

"It's his father's decision. It's been done before, but Dr. Shearer isn't enthusiastic; he suggested they transfer David to another institution."

"Mother, find another way—you're the only one that stands a chance of stopping it."

"Bill, you don't understand, he can't go on—it's a way out for him. Right before the decision, he enlisted my aid to end it all. He's not afraid of death. It's too late—too late to stop the transplant, too late for him. It's been too late for years."

"Mother, I have to trust your judgment, but I don't like it. I don't agree. You're helping to kill him."

Dr. Desmond handed me a letter to read. "Did you know about this?"

Dr. South had written that it was time Baylor did something... but why did she think so? The assistant director of CDP (who had no right to know about the transplant) pointed out that I should have no role in it. The transplant was the "purview of physicians."

As soon as they left, I did what I had wanted to do for weeks: I confided in Jackie. Jackie, horribly shocked, could barely speak.

A week later, Dr. Feigin summoned all involved to a meeting. The conference room was full when I walked in: David's parents, Carol Ann's parents, Father Connelly, three from the Conroe School District, TCH and Baylor public relations, several administrators, Dr. Martin Loren (chief of the medical staff), Dr. Hansen, and another psychiatrist, Susan Thurber, Delores, Marla, and Martha. David's grandmother, relieved to see a familiar face, stood up. "Hi, Mary!" Then Jackie came. The two empty chairs were far apart so we couldn't sit together.

Dr. Feigin spoke first; pointing out that everything said had to remain confidential. He said that on Friday, October 21, David would receive an unmatched bone marrow transplant from his sister. Katherine's surgery would be in Boston. A private jet would fly Carol Ann, Katherine, Sergeant Beeman from security, Dr. Shearer, and his lab assistant to Boston. The jet would remain ready to return Dr. Shearer and the treated bone marrow to Houston. The others would return by commercial flight. Arrangements had been made for them to depart the plane before it reached the gate to avoid any possible reporters.

Dr. Feigin stressed that no one wanted the news media in front of the hospital during the transplant. He conceded that "with such elaborate arrangements and so many people involved, maintaining secrecy will be a remarkable feat." Thursday night, the CRC would be closed and guarded by security.

Dr. Feigin deferred to Dr. Shearer. He said that the Boston researchers who had government approval for limited use of their highly experimental monoclonic antibody treatment of unmatched bone marrow had put forth two conditions: The marrow would be processed by them in their laboratory, and their role would not be made public.

"The marrow will be slowly extracted from Katherine's pelvic bone while [she is] under a general anesthetic," said Dr. Shearer. "I do not anticipate any problems other than weakness and a sore hip. The bone marrow, after treatment with antibodies to clone out the mature T-cells, will be reduced to approximately one-tenth the original volume, and they will be transfused intravenously into David. Hopefully, they will establish residency and provide him with an immune system. David will be given antihistamines and acetaminophen to relieve the expected mild symptoms of a temperature, muscle cramps, and headache. The transfusion itself will take ten minutes."

Dr. Shearer succinctly outlined the four possible outcomes:

In three months to a year, David's immune system would be reconstituted.

An immediate adverse allergic reaction would necessitate taking David out of the isolator and placing him in intensive care.

Other than a slight rash and fever, there should be no graft-versus-host disease. If by chance it did develop, David would be given additional antibodies to remove the few remaining killer cells.

Nothing would happen, in which case David's system would be suppressed by chemotherapy and total body irradiation prior to a second transplant. He intended to explain the procedure and possible complications in detail to David.

All this time looks passed between Feigin, Jackie, and me. Jackie, ashen gray, stricken and immobilized except for eye movement; sick, sick. Feigin and me, ghost white. Each knew the other was envisioning the prolonged suffering of the irradiated leukemia children we had worked with—emaciated, with no hair and distended stomachs. The meeting droned on as the attorney spoke of legal aspects. The school people stated that they would furnish a teacher for three months. After that, David's education would be the responsibility of the hospital teacher.

When everybody got up, Jackie and I made a beeline for each other, but Carol Ann's mother stopped me. Expressing concern over her daughter's weight loss and severe stress, she wanted reassurance that I would be with David while Carol Ann was in Boston.

Back at CDP, I went straight to Jean Alt, R.N., our coordinator. "Clear my schedule for Friday, the twenty-first."

She came to me, steadied me, and asked what was wrong. "Nothing. Just clear my schedule on the twenty-first."

She said one of my appointments coordinated with other clinics and could not be canceled.

I lost my cool and demanded, "Cancel! I can't be here!" Then I stormed out.

Jackie phoned. "Thank you for giving me a week's notice—if I hadn't had time to prepare myself, I would have passed out in that meeting. What about Dr. Feigin's face?"

"Worse than yours. When Shearer said the Boston group demanded anonymity, my stomach went thud. I'm taking vacation next week—this is when I was going to Singapore."

Judy Rozelle, my colleague, did not work on Fridays, so I called her at home. "A big favor, and no questions please. Would you come in on Friday the twenty-first and test one child for me? I have to be with David. Please don't say anything to anybody, just come in and test." She graciously agreed.

Saturday, when my dearest friend arrived to take me to dinner, I couldn't stop pacing.

"What is wrong?"

I wailed, "I can't make it! I can't do it! I'm falling apart!" He said, "I know Bill's fine—it's David?"

"Yes. I'm not God. I can't go through with this."

For the first time in our long relationship, he spoke harshly. "Shut up! Quit pacing. Sit down and hear me. I don't care what you have to do. It's all right for you to carry on—rant and rave and keep on agonizing, but I'll tell you one thing: I know you. In thirty years, I've never seen you fail in a crisis. When the time comes, you will do whatever you must for the boy. He needs you, you'll be there, and you won't falter. Put on your shoes and we'll go eat."

At that moment, his confidence in me made little difference, but later I remembered and his words gave me strength.

My last visit to David's home before the transplant was on Friday, October 14. Everything was set for the next Friday. Both children knew that Katherine was to be the donor. David said, "I'd really rather it had not been her. She's so little. She might be afraid. And anyway, I'm not sure whether I want any of her cells. Do me a favor, please talk to Katherine and see how she really feels."

Katherine said, "It's all right with me, but will they make me take off my underwear on the operating table?"

"Probably, but you'll have a gown on. They'll be very careful not to embarrass you." Her other concern was the possibility of missing the Friday night football game. She had a date with the captain.

David was satisfied when I related her comments, but continued to awfulize over the transplant. We repeated past conversations:

"Why should I have the transplant? Why do you think I should have it? Why are you asking me to agree? If it was you instead of me, what would you do?"

"Quit asking questions—give me a chance to answer. If it were me, not you, it would be the same. My love, I cannot separate myself from you. I would never do something or be a part of something that would hurt you."

"Yeah, I know all that, and that's why if I say no, you will go along with it and say no, too."

"True, but you really don't want to say no."

"I don't know what to expect. What if I panic?"

"Put panic to rest. You will know exactly what is going to happen." "You mean we will have control? It's experimental. What can happen?

I'm not even sure they are leveling with me."

"You're right. It's experimental and therefore we can't be certain of exactly what can or will happen. Dr. Shearer will explain everything he knows to you."

"Well, we haven't done too well talking before. I think it won't work." "You may be right. I understand it is possible that nothing will happen, and it won't reconstitute you."

"That's what I think—I'll go through all this, so will Katherine, and for nothing. All I know is I don't think it will work. What if it does work? What then?"

"That is something you'll have to discuss with Dr. Shearer, but I think it would be a gradual transition: first a sterile room where everybody gowns up, and then home. Only a few people would be allowed around you for a while."

"No matter what, you are saying it won't be easy." "Right."

"Well then, you tell me—Why should I agree to it?" "It's a risk, but if we never dare to risk, we never gain.

All, or most all, meaningful things in life involve risks. Even close relationships always involve risk."

"Not ours." "Oh, yes."

"Why?"

"When we decided to be friends, we both risked being hurt if something happened to separate us."

"Not us—you're wrong."

"No, you took a risk by letting me in your life. I took a risk, too. I knew someday I would lose you—lose you to health or death. Both of us risked being hurt and lonely."

"Oh, no! Mary, Mary, you would never not be my friend! I think I should say no."

"A lot of this is ridiculous. You seem to have forgotten about our conversation last summer."

"Yeah, that was different. I made that decision."

"If you say no and really mean it, your father and Dr. Shearer will not force you." We were quiet for a while.

"Let's play hide-and-go-seek," he said.

Sunday night I awoke in a panic, terrified and certain I was dying. My God, I thought. I've forgotten how to breathe. Afterward, wringing wet, all I could think of was, What if this happens during the transplant? The next night I had another anxiety attack followed by a fear of going back to sleep.

I discussed my experience with my physician, William Obenour. He concluded that it was indeed an anxiety attack.

"You know what it is?" I hesitated. "Probably—I wish for an instant death for David. How can I live if I want him to die? But the foreboding, the specter of him emaciated, suffering a slow death like the cancer kids, just won't go away. This sounds omnipotent—but if I can't make it, David can't."

"I thought it was something like that. The most important thing is to get sleep," he said calmly." You can't go into this without sleep. I'll give you sleeping pills that won't make you groggy—start tomorrow night."

I never took one. Just having the bottle at my bedside was all I needed.

David returned to the hospital on Tuesday morning, October 18. At the CDP, Dr. Shearer emphatically reiterated the need for confidentiality. I cited David's request: No cameras. But if there must be, then have James de Leon from TCH.

"No," Dr. Shearer replied. Baylor has demanded coverage, and they are handling all the arrangements. If the cameras become a problem, or David is compromised, they will be requested to cease."

Dr. Desmond mandated, "After the transplant, the psychiatrist will start seeing David."

Within an hour, everyone seemed to know about the transplant.

Dr. Shearer examined David and, in Carol Ann's presence, fully explained the procedure and answered all of David's questions. Carol Ann was very upset that Dr. Shearer divulged the possibility of serious complications.

Afterward, David told me, "Dr. Shearer and I had a good talk. At least we got some control over the cameras. Now, all the details on the Big Meeting. Who was there? What did you wear? What did Dr. Feigin say?"

"He asked everyone in the room to introduce themselves and briefly state their role."

"Oh, my God! What did you say? You didn't say 'friend'? Friend is not professional."

" 'I support David,' were my words."

"That was good, very good." But then he began awfulizing. "What if I panic with the cameras going and all the strangers?"

"Quit it. This is no different than drawing blood, and I'll be here and you'll be in complete control."

"How can you be so sure?"

"Because I know you, and I know what you can do. After all, you are the star of the show."

Tuesday night he pleaded, "Please stay until I go to sleep, and come early in the morning and drink your coffee here. One more promise—don't leave for one second until after all the critical periods."

That evening his parents and Katherine had visited. Wednesday morning, Carol Ann, Katherine, and Dr. Shearer came in to tell him goodbye before leaving for Boston. While I drank coffee, David instructed, "Double check with the dentist, make sure he'll cover that black line tomorrow afternoon. Why did the lab have to goof on your new cap?"

"Dr. McDaniel thinks we're both nuts—you for thinking my tooth will show in a photograph and me for goin' along with it."

"Mary, you have to look nice. Wear a pretty red dress. Jim says red photographs best."

At noon, his orders continued: "Have you decided on a dress? No gaps down front. Think—what do you have? Maybe you should hit Ella Pryor's for something new. It's a good thing I made you get your hair trimmed last week; it looks good. Don't forget to bring all your makeup. You'll need repairs." On and on he went. I was pleased that he was focusing on trivialities like my appearance, rather than on the procedure and possible complications.

19.

THE TRANSPLANT

"Mary, the evening before the transplant, when you walked in with your suitcase, did you think it would be like this? Me in this crap—out of isolation, sick, and no one knowing what the hell went wrong?"

"That evening I never thought beyond the transplant itself. I put the next day, week, and year out of my mind. The past four months are a blur."

I thought, Thursday, October 20, 1983, seems like years ago. Or was it just yesterday?

The CRC wing was still in operation when I arrived at 7:15 p.m. and I stashed my suitcase under the crib. David said, "No, put it in the room reserved for you, the one with a nice bed. I want you to sleep on the comfortable bed—not on a mat on the floor."

"I planned to sleep in here with you—we'll both sleep better if we are together."

"No. No. You sleep on the comfortable bed."

"Okay. I'll leave the suitcase here until the people clear out."

"Put the suitcase up on the table. We'd better check it right now. If something's not right or missing, you'll have time to go back home. Let's see, red silk blouse with a high collar. That button is in the back. Right? Comb and makeup. Is this jogging suit to sleep in? You did good."

In a lighthearted, almost giddy mood, we talked, watched TV, and played hide-and-go-seek.

The treating of the bone marrow was expected to take six to eight hours, which meant Dr. Shearer would be back around six on Friday morning. David and I were to sleep from 10:00 p.m. until 4:00 a.m., but at 9:00 p.m. Dr. Shearer called. The process had gone quickly and he was leaving for the airport. The transplant would take place around three in the morning.

A flurry of activity followed. Delores cleared the room to make way for the medical equipment. The nurses, Marla and Martha, made last-minute checks and notified people. When they started to disconnect the supply bubble, I told David I was going to bathe and I'd be back in ten minutes. As I stepped out of the shower, Martha came in. "He panicked. He noticed your suitcase gone and thinks you moved to your room. Quick, get back!" I did.

"Mary, where were you? Why did you leave me? You said you'd sleep in here!"

"David, settle down. I'm not moving. I'm not leaving. I had to get my suitcase out of the way." Just then he noticed my ultraconservative gold dressing gown and plopped down on the floor of the crib, moaning. "Oh my God! Mary, look at you! For heaven's sake, get dressed!"

When I returned, he yelled, "You can't wear gold slippers! Don't you know people will be here and cameras going? Three days I've worked on you—put on those pretty black shoes!" He sent me back for minor revisions three times and finally announced, "Now you pass inspection. What a mess you'd be if I hadn't taken charge!"

At midnight all was ready. Marla said, "You two have one hour to rest." I rolled up an exercise mat into a jellyroll, making it exactly the height of the playroom floor. We lay side by side with our heads touching the Plexiglas at the same spot. We had to sit up and stick our faces in the glove to talk. David said, "I don't think we can go to sleep."

"Agreed, but we need to rest."

We lay in silence until Martha, thinking we were asleep, came in quietly. "Time to get up." We got up, the doors opened, and it was "on stage" —two cameramen, father and his best friend Ben, grandparents, public relations, security, and two hospital administrators.

The nurses readied the IV, and Dr. Larry Jefferson, head of the critical care unit, and Dr. Howard Rosenblatt, Dr. Shearer's associate, set up the monitors.

At 1:30 a.m., all four grandparents came in to visit and I went out. Very quickly, Carol Ann's father came after me, saying, "He's getting upset; you have to get back in there."

David, agitated, berated me. "Well, you really goofed up when you left me! You promised you wouldn't leave."

"But your grandparents want to visit with you." "That doesn't make a difference. You weren't here."

At 2:00 a.m., we received word from the airport—the plane was landing, the police escort ready, and they'd arrive in twenty minutes. David sat on the floor of the crib with his back against the port to the playroom with his low table across his lap. In this position, two pairs of gloves, on each side of him, were available to the medical staff.

The cameras started rolling as David's arm and hand were taped to an IV board. For one moment, he became upset because he couldn't see me. He gagged on the liquid Benadryl and Tylenol. After the IV was hooked up, I held the IV pole (the toy rake from the playroom). Holding my arm high became tiring, so Delores took over while I found a stool to stand on.

A beaming Dr. Shearer walked in holding a white Styrofoam ice chest. "Hello, David. Mary, here it is." While Delores uncapped the port, Dr. Shearer gently rotated the plastic bag of fluid that looked like pink lemonade. He placed it in the port. Delores recapped and sprayed in acid. Because I was so close, I got a full dose of acid overspray. As I leaned back, my shoe fell off.

"Oops." David looked at me inquiringly. "My shoe fell off."

"Your shoe fell?" He lowered his head so the camera wouldn't catch his lips; turned up his eyes toward the cameras, and hissed out of the corner of his mouth, "Get it back on!" Dr. Rosenblatt retrieved it and slipped it back on me.

After Delores finished retaping the outside cap, she took over the IV pole. I moved to the window side of the crib and put my hand in the single glove to touch David's leg. The bone marrow bag was sprayed and placed directly into the port of the bubble David occupied. Not having the double protection of two sealed ports between him and the outside worried him. He also didn't trust the oxygen tubes and EKG leads coming in around the edges of the corks on the port caps. During the twenty-minute wait for the acid to sterilize the bag, there was mostly silence. David asked Dr. Shearer, "How is Katherine?"

"Fine—"

I asked, "Did you get any sleep?" "Yes, on the plane."

"You're better off than David and me. We didn't sleep." Standing between Dr. Shearer and Marla when the inside cap was taken off, I was in the logical position to be handed the marrow, but I did not want to touch it. I offered my glove to Dr. Shearer and told David I didn't have a glove. He said,

"That's all right. Just being here is enough. I hope they were all on the level with me about this transplant. Mary, do you know what we're going to do when this is over? Sleep!"

Dr. Shearer took the bag from Martha and gently rotated it while David assisted Marla in placing the EKG leads and the blood pressure sleeve. As Marla inserted the marrow needle into the existing IV on David's wrist, he warned, "Don't stick through!"

After the marrow bag hung on the pole, David repositioned himself. Not once did he hesitate, nor did he wince any time during the transfusion. When bright camera lights shone in David's face, he yelled, "Please stop!"

Dr. Shearer said, "Sorry, David, we have to."

At all times during the infusion my eyes were glued to David or to where he was looking. The silence in the room made the blowers sound deafeningly loud. I had determined that my cognitive processes, not my emotions, would guide my every movement. There would be no gesture or look that David or others might interpret as fear, no startle reaction if something went wrong. Several times when David's breathing seemed quick, I slowly brought my hand up to my chest and he took deep, even breaths. I was so proud of him. He was behaving perfectly.

Toward the end of the infusion, Dr. Shearer, visibly pleased at David's splendid composure, inquired, "How are you doing, David?"

"All right."

At 3:10 a.m., the infusion complete, David became groggy and his head nodded. I had forgotten the two cameramen who alternated being in the room. A moment after a posed picture was taken of the three of us, Dr. Shearer noticed his dark blue suit jacket. "My lab coat! I forgot!" and laughed.

David pretended shock and shook his head, "Too late now."

"You were magnificent," I told David. "A true star." David, drowsy, laid his head on the table and instantly fell asleep. I moved to the other side of the bubble so that I could be closer to him, and Marla laid him back on a pillow. The cameraman came to get a close-up shot of his face, which had fallen into a ghastly repose, mouth wide open. I snapped to, yelling, "No!" and positioned myself between David and the cameraman. I looked pleadingly at Shearer.

"That's enough," he said. The cameraman left. Never again did David have his picture taken.

They woke David every fifteen minutes for vital signs and each time he complained of a headache. I thought he looked awful, but could tell by the faces of the three physicians that all was well. At 5:30 a.m. they took the IV out and he was more comfortable. I sat on a stool with my head on a pillow on the crib baseboard, so that if he awoke, he would immediately see my face. I was in this position when an exuberant Dr. Feigin entered. He grinned and bounced around like a happy kid. "It's a perfect day. The critical periods are over. I must call Jackie." He came back, "I told her he's fine."

"You should be proud of us. Not one hitch. Even so, for some reason, I feel like crying," I said.

Puzzled, he asked, "Why would you want to cry? Everything is great!" He gave me a hug and a kiss and took off, but returned several times.

At 8:00 a.m. they woke David to take vital signs and told him his grandparents would like to come in. But he didn't want to see anybody, and they respected his wishes. He did send them messages: "I love you. I'm fine."

While David supervised reconnecting the supply bubble, I went into the hall and saw Jackie talking to the guard, who wouldn't let her pass. I flew to her and we embraced. "They woke him for vital signs at eight—he's got a headache and is in a foul mood. I wish he'd go back to sleep," I said. David, happy in Jackie's arms, gave me welcomed relief. After Jackie left he cuddled in my arms and watched cartoons. He ordered me to call my mother and tell her we were okay.

David continued to be cantankerous and irritable. He started at any movement or sound and wanted the doors closed for "peace and quiet," but one had to remain partly open.

During the blood drawing at ten-thirty, the nurses, alarmed at seeing two women looking up at the window, said, "There's a leak. They know about the transplant."

I couldn't see because I was in the gloves away from the window, but David looked. "That's Judy and Jean."

I said, "It's okay. They know I'm up here. They're just waving." David inquired, "Judy doesn't work on Friday. Why is she there?"

I said, "She came in to test my kid. I told her I had to be with you."

"Oh! Judy did that for us?" (It was a statement he would repeat many times.) "We'll call her. Tell me exactly what you both said."

All of a sudden I was starving and vexed. Why didn't someone think to bring me food? Everyone was running around happy and excited; we were in this room forgotten. It was ridiculous of me to be angry—any number of people gladly would have brought me food had I asked. I guess I wanted nurturing. After stewing around awhile, I phoned Mildred, and she brought me breakfast from the cafeteria.

Carol Ann and Katherine phoned at a time when David's head "hurt awful." They argued. I didn't know the reason, but David worried. "I'm in trouble—she's going to talk to me when she gets here."

His father, generous with his praise, came in several times. Then he came in very upset. Carol Ann had called again—Katherine wasn't doing well, her lips were blue, she had passed out when she stood up, and she might need a blood transfusion. David Sr., in and out, in and out, was beside himself with worry. Befuddled, David didn't understand and thought Katherine was dying. Ben came in saying he'd made arrangements for a private jet to fly them to Boston. They were ready to leave when Carol Ann called—Katherine was better.

David's headache eased some, but didn't go away. He told the nurses early in the morning that it was gone because "I'm tired of their asking." Alone again, he cuddled in silence and finally said, "Some conversation—Mary, we've done better on the phone. What a lousy day. Let's try again to call Joy."

His father left, and at noon, David agreed to take a nap with me. We lay alongside each other, he on the playroom floor and me on the rolled-up mat. He slept for thirty minutes until they woke him for the vital signs. He ate lunch, we lay down again, and he slept another half hour.

David, less irritable after the second nap, bathed and allowed the grandparents to come in for a few minutes. Around three, his paternal grandmother returned. He chatted with her and gave me permission to leave for ten minutes.

"You got out?" said Jackie, amazed.

"His paternal grandmother is with him."

She remarked, "If he would let anybody in, it would be her. The bubble has never intimidated her; she's just a natural grandmother."

With mixed feelings, watching the clock, David anticipated his mother's arrival. He wanted to see for himself that Katherine was well and had much to tell his mother, but he dreaded "the talk on being ungrateful and disrespectful." He stated, "My mother is supposed to stay tonight, but that doesn't mean you leave—right? If she's here, her friends will come, the phone will ring, ring, she'll talk, talk—my peace and quiet will be gone, and I need it. If you stay here, they'll go to another room."

The story of the transplant made all three network news programs, plus the local stations. David watched, intensely interested, and took issue with some of the reporting, including the characterization of the transplant as "a simple ten-minute procedure."

"Mary," he said, "See why I had to take charge of you? I knew you wouldn't think about your hair and clothes and all, and then, when you saw yourself on TV or your picture in the paper, you'd be sorry."

While we watched the news, Carol Ann and Sergeant Beeman came in arm in arm. Sergeant Beeman asked, "Davey, how are you? Katherine and your mother are fine." And he planted a kiss on Carol Ann's cheek. David, looking both horrified and angry, turned to me and whispered, "Indecent!" Actually, it was comical—Sergeant Beeman, a great big teddy bear, and petite, elegant Carol Ann. For years, the sergeant had taken on an affectionate, fatherly, protective role toward both Carol Ann and David.

"Thank you for being with my son," said Carol Ann graciously. "I wanted to be with him, but if I couldn't, I wanted you to be with him."

I tried to head off her talk with David. "He had absolutely no sleep last night and only two brief naps today. They take vital signs every thirty minutes. He doesn't feel well; he has a headache—it's been a very rough day, but he's been magnificent." If she had really looked at him, she would have known. His face was strained; his usually sparkling eyes were dull and had dark, dark circles under them.

Not deterred, she stated, "I'm not going to tolerate his disrespect."

I tried again. "This isn't the time." But she was determined. I left the room.

David called to me to come back. Carol Ann was talking to her husband on the phone. After hanging up, she said, "My husband would rather have been in Boston with his angel than here. But it was only right that I be with my daughter. I'm very tired. I have houseguests to attend to and feel that I should see that they have a meal. Also, I have many phone calls to make. Would you mind staying tonight?"

After I had agreed and she had left, David looked at me, smiled, and said "Mary, do you realize that you have been standing here for twenty-three hours?" It was now my turn to be irritable. Everything and everybody annoyed me. Totally exhausted, I felt dizzy and realized I should have eaten. It was too late to call someone. I ate a can of David's meat sticks that were slated for a cylinder. About then, a nurse came in raving over the pizza Ben had brought them. David said, "See? Everybody forgets us."

At nine, I took a much needed hot bath and almost immediately dropped off to sleep on a mat under and between the crib and supply. The next morning, David said, "You know, right after you laid down and went to sleep, a nurse came in and looked at you and got real upset—she thought you were dead because you were so plopped out. Your hair is standing straight up and going in all directions—a total mess. You'd better get dressed and get your face and hair fixed before the doctors get here."

When I returned he whimpered, "Now that you're all dressed it doesn't mean you're going to leave, does it?"

"No. I'll stay awhile."

The guard stationed outside David's door called, "Honey, your picture and your name are on the front page of the *Houston Chronicle*. It's time they released your name. You're Dr. Murphy—not another woman." That tag had appeared on previous press photos of David and me together.

I held the paper up against the bubble for David to read. He screeched, "What the hell! What's that mean? 'Pediatrician Murdina Desmond says David wants to walk on grass when he leaves the bubble.' I don't want to walk on grass. I never even thought of walking on grass. Why did she say that?

What right...? How could she?" After the angry storm abated, he continued to read but got upset again. "She says I'm glad. She doesn't know how I feel. She doesn't know me or anything."

Then he turned on me nastily, "You like your picture in the paper, don't you?"

"David, my picture with you has been in the paper lots of times, but my name is with this one, and I think it's a nice picture."

"You like your picture in the paper! You like the attention! You like to be in the center and middle of everything that goes on!"

My first impulse was to lash out, "You demanding brat," but I looked at his quivering lips and the tears on his cheeks; I knew he hated being so dependent upon me. "David, let's look at the stock market," I suggested, and we did.

After that, David wanted the news article again and read aloud the quote of Dr. Shearer:

"We have no experience to use as a gauge. If all goes as well as we envision, I would hope that he could be back at home and starting outside activities within six months."

"People reading this and listening on TV are gonna' forget the words 'experimental' and 'maybe' or 'moderately' before 'optimistic' and think I'm cured." His prediction later proved to be correct.

Drs. Feigin and Shearer checked on David and discussed the ten o'clock press conference. Dr. Desmond came and told David, "I thought I should talk to you. The reporters will ask me questions."

I walked out with her to ask, "Why did you make the comment about his wanting to walk on grass? He wants to know."

"When they started asking for anecdotes," she said, "I remembered your telling me of trying to explain walking in rain puddles and wet grass."

David cried when I said I was leaving. "Your grandparents will be here in a minute, and your mother says they're all going to stay with you through the evening," I said, but he did not seem reassured.

Sunday evening, and thereafter every other evening and always Saturday night, David and I were back to our old routine—current events, my day, the stock market, Westheimer, and hide-and-go-seek. During the day, Jackie and

I both dropped in often, and she visited each afternoon at half past three. He loved our ceaseless hovering. I had coffee with him each morning and usually wrote reports in his room late in the afternoon.

Jackie and I both rushed to stay ahead of our workload—as if we knew of some imminent happening and dared not fall behind.

Dr. Shearer checked each morning and found no evidence of rash, fever, or pain—the first signs of graft-versus-host disease. Three days after the transplant, both Drs. Feigin and Shearer stated they were certain David would not reject. I expressed my relief to Dr. Shearer and shared my panic experiences before the transplant.

"I too had my anxieties. It is an awesome thing we are doing to a life."

The public and the relatives continued to be euphoric—caught up in the "miracle"—and spoke of when, never if, David would come out. David, Jackie, Shearer, and I remained less optimistic. The watching and waiting period strained us.

David constantly looked for a rash on his chest and had me check his back. One evening he exclaimed, "Oh! Look! Look, I got a rash!"

I checked the red line across his chest, "No, that's a mark from leaning against the table edge."

"A rash is red. This is red. Stop laughing. What's so funny?"

"Oh, love, I should have realized that you've never seen a rash and don't know what you're actually looking for." When one of Dr. Shearer's trainees asked David how he felt about his possible cure, he looked at me, "Mary, what's that word for how I feel?"

"Ambivalent."

"That's it. Ambivalent."

When the doctors left, he asked, "What's ambivalent mean?" "Two contradictory feelings at the same time."

"That's it, exactly. Ambivalent."

David loved the attention from Dr. Feigin and liked to remind everyone that Dr. Feigin was the big boss. Jackie once commented, "There is nothing this kid doesn't know about the hierarchy around here. It's interesting when you stop to think of it. I guess the closest thing you could compare it to for the average kid would be a priest, some kind of religious figure, or school principal. In David's case, the ultimate authority figure turns out to be a physician.

If Dr. Feigin was the number-one favorite hospital visitor, Judy Rozelle was number two. She ate lunch with us several times—he knew she would "be careful to not leave crumbs to attract roaches."

One day, before noon, I asked Judy, "Would you please eat lunch with David? I just can't face him. I'd like to run away."

"Your composure, your appearance—it never occurred to me or anyone that you're under a strain," she said.

David gained weight and looked great except for dry, cracked lips. Before the transplant his lips were dry, but now they were raw, and his arms were sore from the daily blood drawing. The rocking, thumb sucking, and facial tics increased, and he spent a lot of time behind closed curtains in the playroom.

After two weeks, David proclaimed, "The transplant didn't take. I would know if it did. I can tell—her cells are gone."

The next week I asked Shearer if maybe nothing was going to happen. He shook his head. "I don't know. So far everything is too easy. I would be more comfortable if something would have happened."

Jackie and I worried. David was becoming more depressed, and the rush of attention following the transplant was diminishing. Though he did not believe the transplant had worked, we spoke about his coming out of the bubble.

"I'm not sure I can make it," he said fretfully. "It won't be easy," I agreed.

"Do you think I'm so dumb that I couldn't watch someone shampoo their hair one time and then be able to do it?"

"There is not a doubt in my mind you can learn everything you need to learn. I'm concerned that you'll be bombarded with three hundred different things all at once."

"Like what?"

"Like wearing shoes."

"Me, wear shoes? Never. Why should I wear shoes? No, forget it, no shoes."

"Everyone wears shoes. For one thing, you might step on a piece of broken glass. What could happen is that when you came out, you'd step on something and hurt your foot, and a mosquito could land on your face—two new things in one second's time. But we can deal with things if we have a plan so that everything doesn't hit at once."

"Sounds reasonable. But shoes?"

"One step on an ice-cold sidewalk and you'd put on shoes. Seriously, what is the one thing you would like to do?"

"The whole idea is so overwhelming—I just don't know. I just don't know. I guess maybe I'm curious about my room at home—where I'd sleep. Going to a school and dealing with kids will be the big problem."

"We'll have to work on that the most."

"Well, I have nothing in common with anybody my age. What's the point in even trying to deal with anybody my age?"

"You can't and won't want to avoid other kids."

"I could probably make it in an adult world."

"You're probably right. But if you come out, you'll have common interests with kids at school, and you'll feel different about making friends with someone your own age. Our relationship will change. A whole world will open to you. We will always love each other, but you'll have other interests that are appropriate for a teenager. I won't be as important as I am now, but that is right. It's the way it should be. You won't need the kind of relationship we now share."

"Oh, Mary, I'll always need you! Nothing will ever change between us, ever."

David was correct; he had had virtually no experience in dealing with peers. Now, more than ever, Jane and I wanted a friend in addition to Shawn for him, but finding someone seemed impossible until Judy mentioned that her son avidly followed David's life. Andrew, a bright boy... Maybe?

David, happy to have Judy come in the evening, did not object to Andrew, telling me laughingly, "I know you maneuvered this. You want me to relate to someone my own age."

"You don't have a monopoly on manipulation." Andrew's many visits became the bright spot in David's life and provided input from the "real" world of an eleven-year-old.

Surprise of surprises, David became interested in Andrew's *Encyclopedia Brown* books and requested Jackie and I read them aloud. On Thanksgiving Day, Andrew brought a tiny telescope, which, unlike the binoculars that David had, gave a clear view through the PVC. He could see inside cars and the hotel rooms.

For some reason, David kept this possession a secret from the nurses and swore me to secrecy. Maybe he was afraid they would chastise him.

One morning a bright blue-and-red leaded glass football player about six inches high hung from a string attached to a suction cup on the window. I said, "Beautiful..." and reached toward it. He screamed, "Don't touch that! Andrew made it! You might break it."

Judy told me Andrew's feelings were hurt because David didn't talk. She admonished David, "You were rude to Andrew last night."

"I had homework."

"When he called, why didn't you tell him you had homework?"

"If I did that he wouldn't come and I wanted him to come."

I thought if he gets out of here we have a long, long way to go on social skills with peers.

At a meeting on November 14, 1983, Dr. Desmond said that David needed psychiatric counseling to handle any adjustment problems. She also discussed with the nurses ways to deal with David's "boredom." Jackie and I looked at each other and shook our heads in dismay as the discussion became bizarre, far removed from what was going on with David.

Afterward, Jackie described the solidifying relationship between Feigin, Shearer, Carol Ann, herself, and me: "It's a circling of the wagons, a bracing for the impending event, be it good or bad. Our group is closed. Prior to the transplant, a new team member possibly could have been added and accepted, but now as an exclusive, defined group. We will resist any outsiders. This is why I so resent Desmond's insistence on psychiatry."

I, too, bitterly resented it. Psychiatry never helped before, why or how could it do anything now except invade our privacy and add another problem for David? That evening when I walked in David's room, he pointed to me. "You! You work for a fool!"

"What?"

"I told you—you work for a fool. I do not want one more nurse walking in here trying to 'stimulate' me by 'interacting.' If I'm bored, it's because I choose to be bored, and furthermore, I'm not crazy. I'm not going to talk to a shrink."

"You don't have to be crazy to talk to a psychiatrist. You discuss feelings."

"Well, I can't talk to anybody about my feelings."

"That's not true. You talk to me."

"That's different—I can trust you. But if Desmond tells a shrink to see me, then he's gonna tell her what I tell him. And for sure he doesn't care anything at all about me. He's just following her orders."

"No, he wouldn't say what you said. Psychiatrists aren't supposed to; therapy sessions are confidential."

"That's not true. He isn't coming here to see me for any reason except she told him to. And when you're told to do something then you have to report back. She ordered him to see me, so don't try to tell me that he won't tell her."

The psychiatrist came three times a week, but David went into the playroom and drew the curtains. Once, he taped up a note that read: Get the Hell out of here. His mother saw the note and made David apologize.

He inquired, "I know you don't want to get involved in my battle with psychiatry, but who, in your opinion, will last the longest?"

"David, I'm not making any bets, but you've had a lot more experience doing nothing than most people." He steadfastly refused to speak, insisting that the apology his mother had forced him to make would be his only words ever to the psychiatrist.

I wrote virtually all of my reports while with David. He continued to show interest in current events, especially anything on AIDS or child abuse. We watched a TV report of a boy born prematurely who had received AIDS from a blood transfusion. Clearly, this disease was not confined to homosexuals and posed a threat to the general public. My mind was somewhat cluttered during this period, and I had little interest in AIDS; but David, realizing the implications of the lethal virus, forced me to listen and gather information.

We watched a report on patricide in Wyoming. A sixteen-year-old boy and his fourteen-year-old sister ambushed and killed their father with six blasts from a shotgun. The children had reported the beatings and sexual abuse to the school authorities and to the police. The investigative reporter interviewed these officials; all gave the same reason for not believing the children's story—the father, an Internal Revenue Service agent, was a righteous, upstanding man. At the trial, the mother described years of sexual abuse of the girl, and neighbors told of hearing screams.

Afterward, David asked, "How could a father do that? How could a mother know and not stop it? Why didn't the police believe them? Why did they convict and send that teenager to prison?"

Long November finally ended. Forty days since the transplant, and no apparent change at all. David described the days as "more of the same nothing." Jackie and I stood by, helpless, as despondency and malaise enveloped him. On Friday, December 2, the lab work revealed a change, possibly the first cell to be restored. Dr. Shearer, though encouraged, said, "It's too soon to be sure."

Saturday night, David demanded, "Be here Monday night—a real special TV program is on." On Monday evening, December 5, he asked me to leave the room to make my tea. When I returned, he called out, "Happy Birthday! You thought I forgot. Open your present. Like the purse? Let me organize things in the new one."

He should have been happy that the surprise party went as he had planned, but he remained unaccountably somber and often gripped his stomach.

"Does your stomach hurt again?"

"No, it feels funny and I'm tired." Cuddled in my arms, he half-smiled, and as our eyes locked a cold chill went through me—he's dying. I tried to shake the ominous feeling, telling myself that he had an ulcer. The next morning, Dr. Shearer disagreed with my diagnosis, asserting that there was no medical evidence of an ulcer.

At the December CDP meeting, psychiatry described their therapeutic approach and progress. Dr. Desmond expressed pleasure over their success in having established a relationship with David. The adjustment problems were no longer a concern. Jackie and I shook our heads in disbelief and never uttered a word. As we left the meeting, Jackie said, "Why ruin such a glorious report with reality? Strange, when you think about it. No one mentioned to them that David can't hear them through the Plexiglas walls of the playroom."

Each morning Dr. Shearer and I, both inexpressibly weary, mutely looked at each other, but the week before Christmas he said, "After the holidays, I'm going to assign a fellow to David. I can't tolerate seeing him each day. I'm too involved. I'm losing my objectivity. The whole situation takes all my thoughts. It isn't fair to my other patients and my students."

I nodded. "I understand. It's consuming us, isn't it?"

"Yes, it really is. The nights are the really bad time."

We discussed our doubts and second thoughts about everything and our mutual fear of having David out of our sight and forty miles away for several days. I still held to my stress induced ulcer hypothesis. Dr. Shearer still did not know what the progressive change in the cell "markers" in the lab reports signified. David would be going home on Thursday, three days before Christmas. I intended to take vacation from Wednesday until after New Year's Day. But late Tuesday afternoon, Dr. Desmond and I learned that we had to see two abused teenagers—that was the end of my vacation that week.

Wednesday morning, David assumed I came just to have coffee with him.

"No, two consults have to be tested."

"Oh!" he exclaimed. "You're here to see that sister and brother. They're twelve and fourteen. They were brutally abused. The boy's arm is broken and the girl can't walk because her feet were bound with wires. It must be awful. They say the parents tortured them."

He wanted verification of the rumors. That evening I merely said, "What you heard is true. It is awful." I didn't tell him how awful.

After a long silence, he said, "Parents love their children. Why? I don't understand the violence in the world."

"Neither do I."

Andrew spent all day Wednesday with David. David said, "We had a wonderful time."

Thursday morning, Jackie and I saw David off for home. He was somewhat uneasy at being away from Dr. Shearer but was eager to leave. He asked, "Mary, what day will you visit?"

"I'm not. You'll be away only three days, and you'll be busy with Christmas, friends, and family. Lots will be going on."

"But you could still come. I haven't been without you for sixty-seven days."

"Then it's time we break the habit."

Lorna and Bill arrived from Singapore on Christmas Eve, and the holidays were a happy, happy time. Dr. Shearer had little choice but to accept the parents' decision to keep David at home until after New Year's. I talked with David several times on the telephone, and he seemed in good spirits. I concluded that all of my worries over the "stress ulcer" and the specter of death were an overreaction from the strain and exhaustion of these past five months. My son's joy and the coming baby made me hopeful that the pleasure of the holidays would continue into the next year.

20.

THE ER

"This year has been shit," David said. "In more ways than one."

"It's been 109 days since the transplant—one day out of the bubble." "This morning at the Wednesday case conference, everyone was waiting for my report on the historic event. I said you weren't really out of isolation; we now merely enter your new sterile chamber. Indy told them the TV coverage of your exit didn't resemble the one she witnessed."

"Have you heard from Bill? Does he know I'm out?"

"He called his grandmother. He heard it on the Singapore news. He has been calling often, and she says he always asks if I know what's wrong. She tells him I have no idea, and neither does anyone else. He's worried and offered to fly back."

"Two good things—our baby will be here in two months, and that name Jack Miguel is scratched. What if Bill hadn't realized Miguel is the name of a Philippine beer? Imagine a son named after beer. Has he decided on another name?"

"I don't know."

"Call Bill. Tell him this is too important to put off until our baby is born. I want that name settled immediately."

"You made that point clear to him." "I upset Bill."

"Your behavior that night is best forgotten."

David returned to the hospital on Monday, January 2, 1984. He had been looking forward to a visit from Lorna and Bill.

When we arrived, Bill told him that we were famous worldwide. "That transplant picture of you, Mother, and Shearer is every place I go—India, China, Malaysia, and Brunei."

"Brunei, by Borneo, where the richest man in the world lives?" David asked.

Bill answered, "Yes, I've been to the Sultan's palace." David asked Lorna, "What have you been doing?"

"Bill had to go to Colorado on business and I went with him. I saw snow. Did you ever see snow?"

"Yes. Snowflakes are symmetrical." With childlike wonder and delight, Lorna told of rolling in deep snow. David, caught up in her animated description, "rolled in the snow" with her.

David remarked, "I like the name Laura Marie for the baby, but the doctor could be wrong—you need a name for a boy."

"Jack Miguel," Bill proposed. "Jack is simple and Miguel is Filipino." "Jack Miguel doesn't sound right. Start thinking of another name," David commanded.

David, pointing to Lorna's huge stomach, inquired, "How does it feel to carry all that?"

"Heavy," she replied. "I get tired."

David asked Bill and me to leave so he could talk with Lorna. Later, both reported a beautiful encounter. As Lorna put it, "I lifted up my blouse and David put his gloved hands on my belly." With astonishment, David told me of the baby moving.

"I'm hungry," declared Lorna, after we were all back in the room. "David, do you want me to bring you an ice cream?"

"No, thank you. I have three ice creams in my refrigerator." "I didn't know you had a refrigerator."

"Oh, yes, right over there next to my shower."

I was sitting on a little chair close to the transport when David hit my upper arm with his fist.

"That hurt!"

Bill spoke up. "No one strikes my mother. Now listen, kid, I am the one who should be jealous. After all, I've been sharing my mother with you for years, and that's all right because I think of you as my little brother. Apologize. Now do we understand each other?"

Lips quivering and penitent, David apologized. "I'm sorry."

"Fine. Wait 'til Lorna figures out she's been had about the refrigerator and shower. She'll be hot."

After they left for a tour of the hospital, David continued to be sullen and turned down my offer to play hide-and-go-seek.

"What is the matter with you? Does your stomach hurt?"

"No. Listen, did you do as I asked and get everything ready for your tax return? I can't deal with an extension this year."

The next morning, David, kneeling in the crib and rocking, broke down in sobs when he saw me. With the bright morning light on his face, I immediately knew he was ill.

"Oh, love, what's wrong? Does your stomach hurt?"

"I have a fever. It's 99.6. Will you come tonight and stay until I'm asleep?"

At noon I held a pale, listless, ill boy for an hour. That evening, still exhausted, David huddled in my arms to watch TV. Then he lay down and I read to him for over an hour. At ten we turned out the lights. I pressed my hands on his back until he fell asleep at midnight.

Everyone except David and I viewed the low-grade fever with optimism. Surely, the doctors said, it signified mild graft-versus-host disease and the beginning of David's acquiring an immune system. Fear and grief engulfed me. I based my morbid dread on my own stomachaches and his silent eyes. Most alarming to me was his refusal to play hide-and-go-seek. I found myself begging him to play. He didn't say no, he merely shook his head as if to say, Mary, no more fun and games, this is serious. It is over. Looking into his eyes, I saw life fading away. My own stomachaches mirrored the intensity of his—we felt each other's pain.

I saw very little of my son that week. Bill said, "Little Mother, we've had a good visit. Go to David."

Thursday evening, David phoned.

"Will you be here at seven?"

"Yes. I'm almost ready to leave."

He sounded relieved.

"Okay, I was just checking. See ya in a few minutes."

When I saw him pacing and terror stricken, I dropped my coat and purse on the floor in the rush to get in the gloves. Huddled in my arms, he cried, "My temperature is 104!"

Actually, it was 100.4 degrees; he had misheard the nurse. Tylenol quickly brought his temperature down, but the remainder of the week his fever repeatedly shot up to over 100. On Monday it went over 101. The worse he felt, the more he sucked his thumb and rocked. Having never been ill a day in his life, he did not know how to be sick and resisted all suggestions to lie down. "No one lays down in the middle of the day," he said.

That evening David said, "Let's call your mother." In the ensuing conversation, my mother suggested that he should lie down. Once again, she had shown her magical ability to get David to do things. He lay down, dozed, and awoke shivering, but remained down. He remarked, "She's right, it's better laying down. Hold my back."

David's temperature rose above 102 and he complained of a stomachache. Dr. Shearer arrived that night at half past ten. Perplexed, he told me he did not know if it was GVH or an infection.

Bill phoned. "Mother, that boy is really sick. Grandmother said he asked her advice. Now you and Shearer are there in the middle of the night. What is going on?"

All day Tuesday David insisted he felt fine. But that evening, he chilled with a fever of 102.8. He complained of a dry throat, gagged, and spit up the thick Tylenol syrup. It became impossible to know how much Tylenol he actually swallowed.

Lorna and Bill left that morning without my seeing them again. Calling from the airport, Bill asked, "Mother, what is wrong? Don't tell me he won't get well. Is it the transplant?"

"No one knows. Everyone's optimistic that he's being reconstituted. I'm worried about an ulcer. Dr. Shearer is checking for infection—his platelet count fell."

"Mother, you shouldn't have agreed to the transplant. You should have taken my advice, used your energy and influence to get him turned over to

NASA. He could have lived in one of their large chambers and become the perfect astronaut."

"He's feeling better this morning. Maybe I shouldn't be pessimistic."

Distraught when Bill phoned the next morning from California, I lamented, "David's dying, and he knows it."

"Mother, you are wrong. He can't. He's never lived. Don't you dare tell me Little Brother is dying."

"Listen, Bill, please try to understand. I couldn't make your dreams for him come true. I regret the transplant, but last summer it seemed a way out. David decided he could not continue living in a dependent, hopeless state. He knew what he was doing. Making that ultimate choice gave him control and gave him freedom."

"I'm flying back."

"No. Lorna... the baby."

Wednesday, January 11, eighty-two days after the transplant, Dr. Shearer cautiously stated, "David's illness is probably graft-versus-host disease and the beginning of reconstitution."

That afternoon Jackie, Carol Ann, and I sat alongside the transport talking with David. Carol Ann, elated over the latest events, said, "That's your sister's cells working inside of you."

David shot her a dirty look as if to say, "I'm not sure I want her cells working in me." She spent the evening with her son.

David lay down much of the time, and he napped in the playroom while the psychiatrist visited. Thursday, Jackie described David as "looking ghastly, like he really felt sick, but he insisted on sitting up and playing Boggle. By midnight, his fever was over 103. Friday, he complained of stomach cramps, and his stomach was noticeably enlarged.

Saturday night, weak and pale, he coughed from nine until midnight. He murmured, "My stomach feels like it's lost control."

So much happened the week of January 16. Monday morning Dr. Celine Guerra examined David. Dr. Shearer told me he gave a lot of thought to selecting this casual young physician with her easy sense of humor to work with David.

Celine found David "endearing." She recalled how David referred to Dr. Shearer as "old William." As she put it, "Not one of us trainees would ever refer to Dr. Shearer with such familiarity."

That same day, Dr. Shearer termed the significant rise in David's immunoglobulin counts a "significant development that probably meant reconstitution."

He told David and me details of the lab work, but no one could answer David's question: "If I have GVH, why didn't I have the rash first?"

Dr. Shearer ordered two rooms prepared—either for David's transition from isolation or for emergency treatment if his sickness worsened. David followed the remodeling with interest. I made daily reports and drew floor plans.

Every time I encountered Dr. Feigin he exuberantly exclaimed, "Great news! The lymphocytes are up!" and dismissed my protest that David remained obviously ill. Finally, I, too, believed that David was gaining immunity.

As his fever lessened, for two short days David allowed himself to consider the real possibility of getting out of isolation. He asked Jackie to bring her summer vacation photographs back—pictures he had previously politely and briefly scrutinized with no interest. With a wistful look, he asked her to tell him about the mountains and the lakes in the pictures.

I, too, experienced his longing.

"Maybe we will walk up the sidewalk to your house. Would you have a place for me?"

"Yes, love. I always thought my condominium would be a perfect transition place for you. It's near the hospital, very private, and no children."

"Where would I sleep?"

"In my big bed. The bedroom is very large and we could get another bed for your mother. I'd sleep at my neighbor's. It would be perfect." Friday and Saturday the fever stayed down and David seemed fairly comfortable. Early Sunday night he went to sleep cuddled in my arms and awoke saying, "Mary, I feel fine. I'm not sick anymore." His eyes sparkled and he chattered like a magpie.

"You know what your problem is?" he asked me. "Your problem is that you don't have enough social life. You'd have more energy and feel better if you went on dates and had fun at parties."

"Dates and parties take time."

"If you got yourself organized, you'd have time."

"When? I'm either here, working, or sleeping."

"Tell you what—I won't talk while you write reports and you'll finish by four-thirty. Drive home, dress pretty, go have fun, and be back here by seven. All you need is organization."

"Love, you're impossible."

He went to sleep at ten o'clock, listening to the Beatles. I wrote a note in his chart: "Definitely better." I persuaded myself that Dr. Feigin was right, and I was wrong. For the first time in three weeks I slept soundly all night.

But it was right back to despair on Monday morning, the week of January 23. David, very ill, now had a runny nose and constant facial twitches. He insisted the cough and choking were due to something like a feather stuck in his throat. Celine, seeing two nodes, which resembled tonsils in his throat, encouraged my simplistic reasoning—growth of tonsils meant an immune system.

Tuesday afternoon I was staying with David until Jackie arrived. At three-thirty he panicked, "Something's happened to Jackie." I called her office; she was supposedly on her way. He rocked and sucked his thumb—almost out of control. When I told a nurse to page Jackie, she replied, "Oh, Jackie called some time ago and said she wouldn't be here until four." He cried in relief.

About five o'clock Wednesday afternoon we were watching Fannin Street when David said, "I want you to get married."

"Me, get married? Why?" "You should have a husband."

"I like being single."

"That's right, you tried marriage."

"I did indeed. Marriage isn't in my thoughts. Anyway, I don't know a man I want to marry. Nor do I know a man who's ready to propose."

"There are lots of men you can marry. Look down at the parking lot. See all those men. You could marry any one of them."

"That's absurd."

"No. If any one of those men got to know you, they would want to marry you—to love you and take care of you."

"Do you have any idea how wonderful it is to have you believe I'm so special I can marry any man?"

"You could marry any man in the world. I don't want you to live alone. Promise you'll at least give it some thought."

"Promise." As if we didn't have enough problems, a request came from Salt Lake City for Dr. Shearer to perform a bone marrow transplant on T.J., a ten-month-old boy with SCID. Dr. Shearer reviewed the records and told me he thought the case hopeless because of the child's widespread infection. However, political pressure overrode his medical judgment, and on February 1, 1984, the infant was admitted to CRC and occupied what were to have been David's transition quarters. What a cruel blow—Jackie and I knew it was just a matter of time until David had to come out of the bubble, and there was not another set of rooms with a view of Fannin Street.

Carol Ann soon met T.J.'s parents and brought them into David's room. They were teenagers. The father was designated as the donor, and a few nights later he came in to question David about Katherine's surgery—did it hurt?

"There's nothing to it. Besides, you're big, Katherine is little," David reassured him. The baby received his transplant and, in a very short time, his immune system was reconstituted.

Dr. Shearer told me, "It isn't fair. This should have been David."

During the last week in January, David deteriorated rapidly. Monday evening, he would sleep about ten minutes, wake up and look at me for a moment, try to hold his head erect, and doze off again. He was content with my hands pressed against his back.

That night, David was fairly comfortable as we watched TV. Then, suddenly, he started chilling. I had just gotten him covered with the Big Bird blanket and socks on his hands when the nurse came to take vital signs. She read the thermometer—over 104—and sternly lectured, "Why wasn't I called?" David shook his head; I tried to explain that it all happened in one minute, but she wasn't appeased.

Thursday morning, February 2, David was desperately ill—constipated and choking. That night, the nurses termed David's condition as "acute distress." His fever was above 105 and he could hardly breathe. I read *Encyclopedia Brown* until my voice was gone.

Friday afternoon, Jackie and I faced a shattered David. "My mother looked at me and ran out—she got into the car and drove out." He falteringly whimpered, "She ran away. She'll never come back. We'll never, ever see her again." Jackie or I had to stay with him.

Carol Ann walked in my office and we embraced.

"I looked at David and it wasn't him," she said tearfully. "It was Baby David Joseph dying. I couldn't face it. I ran."

"Jackie and I figured it was something like that. Remember your sessions with Louise Haine back in 1974? She worried then that you hadn't worked through the grief of losing the baby."

"She's right. There just never was time. Please come with me to face my son.

Dr. Shearer came in and requested Carol Ann to come to his office. She asked, "Can Mary come along?"

In the privacy of his office he informed us, "He's going down. And I don't know what is wrong—an infection or GVI. I'm having another set of rooms prepared. I'll probably have to take him out of isolation."

Carol Ann said, "Dr. Shearer, one request please. If you do, make certain Mary is there."

Carol Ann went home that evening. I read to David until two in the morning. Most of the night his temperature remained over 104. One of Dr. Shearer's fellows stayed on CRC all night. Carol Ann spent Saturday, Sunday, and Monday nights at the hospital. David's temperature hovered over 105.

The week of February 6, 1984, was awful. As David's condition worsened, so did my own stomachaches. Monday morning David vomited, but still I tried to feed him. He looked at me and shook his head. Incredibly ill, with a swollen stomach, dry skin, and bleeding lips. He hunched over with his head on folded arms. I recoiled in horror. I saw Bill's powerful painting *Agony* and ran out of the room.

I went to Dr. Feigin's office and demanded, "What is happening? Tell me what's going on. What's wrong with him?"

Putting his arm around me consolingly, he said, "Don't be upset. He'll be fine. His lymphocytes are up."

I pulled away and sharply retorted, "I don't care about his lymphocytes! He's so sick. He won't take one bite of food. Before, he always ate a little just to please me. Now, nothing for two days."

"Mary, I am worried," he confessed. "I'm worried about liquids, not food. He's dehydrated. Forget food—he needs fluids. Get back up there and get him to take fluids."

My fantasy that liquids would be the cure took over. I ran back upstairs and yelled for Potts. "Dr. Feigin says liquids. Which ones?"

She followed me, saying, "He needs salts. Let's try juice from the tuna and ham." He swallowed several sips for me, I wished for an eyedropper to squirt some down his throat.

Tuesday morning, Dr. Shearer told David he might have to come out of the bubble. At noon, David said, "Mary, I feel so terrible. Stay and hold me, and please don't go home tonight. I don't think I can get through the night without you. My mother went home this morning."

"All right. I'll go home after my one o'clock appointment for a change of clothes."

I was throwing things into an overnight bag when Mildred phoned to tell me to call Dr. Shearer immediately. He said, "Mary, how quick can you be here? I'm going to take David out within the hour."

"Five to ten minutes," I said.

"Everyone needed has been notified, and I've spoken to his parents."

I grabbed my half-packed bag and ran to the car, drove fast, and ran from the parking lot to my office. I yelled for Judy, "They're going to take David out! Come with me!" Going out the door, I asked Jean to page Jackie and tell her to get to CRC quick. Judy walked up to CRC and sat with me for a few minutes until I caught my breath. She stayed in the hall after I went in to David.

Jackie arrived and a moment later Dr. Shearer walked in saying, "David, I want to talk to you." He nodded towards us, "I want you two to stay. David, we're going to have to take you out to treat you."

"Well, if you think that's best," David said, surprisingly calm. "But you'd better let my parents know." Dr. Shearer hurriedly left.

David turned to me. "Mary, do I have any immunity at all?"

"You have some. Your lymphocytes are up. We don't know if it's enough or not."

"Well, that will have to do. It really doesn't make any difference anyway. I feel so bad, nothing could be worse."

Dr. Guerra came in. David, rocked, sucked his thumb, and rubbed his forehead like mad. I asked, "Is there anything you would like to take or have? I'll bet you can get a Coke when you're out."

He perked up. "Do you think Potts could do that?" "Maybe. Let's phone and ask her."

With everything ready for David's exit from the bubble, we waited for his parents. But his father arrived in a wild, angry state and asserted, "You aren't going to take my son out!" He came in, spoke to David, then stood in the doorway to the anteroom with his arms braced against the door frame and his feet wide apart, blocking the entrance and screaming, "No! No!"

Dr. Shearer reached out his hand saying, "Now, David, you've got to listen to me. He's going down. There's no choice. Minutes are important. We don't have time."

David Sr. broke down, the anger turned to grief and he pleaded, "Not until his mother's here."

After ten minutes, Dr. Shearer said, "Five more minutes at the most." Carol Ann then arrived, took her husband's arm, and they walked away.

21.

TWO WEEKS OUT OF THE BUBBLE

"Mary, this is all crazy—me like this with all the tubes, me out of isolation and in this room. All I remember about coming out is your face and Dr. Shearer's face. He helped me, didn't he?"

"Yes, he did. You were very weak. It happened too fast to remember."

Dr. Shearer ordered, "I want this done the simplest way." Delores pushed a gurney to the end of the supply bubble. She quickly untaped the outside cap, and David pulled off the inside cap. Dr. Shearer handed him a bio respirator mask. David, in the fetal position, stuck his head out of the port, hesitated, and drew back.

I said, "Love, it's all right, I'm right here." Dr. Shearer reached up and put his hands under David's shoulders and gently lifted him out.

Over the years I had often imagined this moment, the moment when David would leave the bubble. Yet here it was, actually happening, and it would be headline news all over the world, but I felt nothing. It was just another event in the one staggering moment of disbelief and grief that was January and February.

David quickly pulled the sheet over his head, and we wheeled him down and across the hall to his new room. At the door I said, "I won't leave. I'll sit right by the door. If you need anything, call me." The transfer had taken only a few seconds. I glanced at my watch—3:20 p.m., February 7, 1984.

Jackie and Judy joined me. Judy turned white on hearing our wishes for David. "Let him go quickly," Jackie said.

"Don't let him live long," I said.

Dr. Donald J. Fernback, head of hematology, awaited David to immediately withdraw a bone marrow sample. Sensibly, Ruth Sylvester, director of TCH nursing, ordered Marla to be in the room so David would see a familiar face. Meanwhile, David's mother, father, and sister were readying themselves in sterile gowns, facemask, cap, and gloves to go into his room.

Dr. Shearer walked up to me. "We're taking David down to X-ray. They've spent over an hour sterilizing the room. Security is clearing the way. Gown up and let's go."

I quickly donned the sterile garb and waited for David to be wheeled out. David took one look around, and then again, pulled the sheet over his head. We ran fast down the hall as if to escape all the germs in the world. Time was critical in diagnosing David's illness, and we were holding up the line of patients in X-ray.

A bystander approached, "What's going on?"

I held up my hand. "You don't want this disease!" I barked, and he backed away.

David poked his head out and with amazement said, "A breeze!" Shivering, with teeth chattering from his temperature rising over 105, he lay on the cold metal X-ray table. I enfolded him in my arms. Having him in my arms without the gloves was a tender moment, but my only thought was to keep him warm. He asked what the barium tasted like. The radiologist had said peppermint ice cream. "What is peppermint?"

Between X-ray shots, I held him. From behind the shield I could view the TV monitor; someone said, "No ulcers."

Back upstairs, David said, "Hurry, Mary, and get re-gowned so you can come in."

Intravenous antibiotics, gamma globulin, and nutrients made David feel better. His mother combed his hair and doted over him. I sat in the chair, mostly silent. Katherine sat on the sink with her feet on the bed. I thought about how many billion germs were on her shoes. (The next day, we wore booties over our shoes.)

David repeatedly remarked, "This bed is soft. Marla says it's not a waterbed." Katherine explained the control panel. David commented, "I didn't know there were so many things in the world."

I was totally unprepared for the difference in David's voice. Out of the bubble, he spoke loudly and sounded like a man. The high pitch disappeared.

Probably his speaking loudly to overcome the blower noise had heightened his pitch, or possibly the drone of the motors had masked the low range of his voice. By the next day, adjusted to the absence of the blowers, he spoke at a normal conversational level. A second shock occurred when I saw him nude during various testing procedures. He was clearly becoming sexually mature. David was no little boy.

Outside the bubble, David had a primitive startle reaction to virtually any movement or sound. When Katherine sat with her feet on his bed, chatting away, she waved her arms, and he recoiled as if to avoid being struck.

When David's father came in, I left to make phone calls. At eight in the evening I went back. His father said, "Mary, go home, you need rest. You're tired from three nights at the hospital. I'm staying tonight."

David piped up, "Mary's staying. She promised this afternoon." David Sr., not a man for sitting and doing nothing, was in and out of the room all during the night.

Around nine o'clock, Dr. Shearer and I were alone with David. His fever shot up over 105, and Dr. Shearer handed David a large white Tylenol tablet.

David looked at it in bewilderment. Dr. Shearer urged, "Go ahead, take it." David, in utter desperation, looked at me.

"There is no way he can swallow that pill," I said. "He's never had anything solid in his mouth in his life. Besides that, his mouth is dry and his throat is closed." From then on I became the pill crusher. Even then, he could hardly swallow the powdered Tylenol mixed with water.

The Tylenol incident over, David announced he had to have a bowel movement. Dr. Shearer declared, "Let's go." The IV fluids had miraculously restored some of David's strength, but he was still weak and unaccustomed to walking a distance of more than five feet. I was ready to give up and yell for a bedpan before we started, but Dr. Shearer persisted.

David, with both wrists taped to IV boards, couldn't manage to sit up without help. Sitting on the edge of the bed, feet dangling, he became frightened and wanted me to hold him tight. After he stood on the floor, his fear of falling left. Dr. Shearer and I had to contend with a weak, awkward, perplexed boy and two IV poles. We mistakenly got him out on the far side of the bed, which entailed more steps to the bathroom.

We finally got to the door and I laughed. "How do three of us and two poles get through this door, and then, where do we stand after we're in? This should be filmed and sold as the comedy of the year!" I considered. "I'll go first, stand in the bathtub and pull the two poles in and then you two come in. David, I'll turn my back after I get the poles situated."

I couldn't see, but heard what was going on. David, with immobilized hands, could not pull down his shorts and objected to any assistance. Then, in alarm, he blurted out, "We forgot the washcloths!"

"Washcloths? What for?" asked Dr. Shearer.

"Washcloths to clean me."

"Use toilet tissue."

"Who me? Not me. Never. It's not sterile."

"You have no choice, you have to use the tissue."

"No, not me."

"But you have to."

Finally, I broke in. "David, there's no choice—not a one of us can move. Use the toilet tissue, it's a new, sterile roll, and then when you're back in bed, I'll fix two sterile washcloths with sterile water, and you can use them as usual."

At ten o'clock, I showered and put on a jogging suit. Having no slippers or socks for my cold feet, I took a pair of David's socks from the bubble. I was lying on the cot when he noticed.

"What do you have on your feet?" he asked.

"A pair of your socks."

"I was afraid of that. How did you get them?"

"Simple, I reached in the supply bubble where you came out and took them."

"Make certain you put them right back where you got them, tomorrow."

"Don't worry. I'll not keep your holey socks, but tonight I'm not going around barefooted with freezing feet."

David, constantly choking, could not get rid of the mucus in his mouth, so I had to clean out his mouth with a damp washcloth. I kept thinking that something was wrong, something was different, but what? I finally realized—

he had not put his thumb in his mouth since he left the bubble. He wanted me to look at his arm. One glance and I reeled back, stunned—Dr. South's white skin graft had turned red and seemed to be rising, blistering. After twelve years, was he rejecting her patch of skin?

When he was notified, Dr. Feigin said, "Amazing. That graft lay dormant for twelve years."

All night was busy, busy—medications, tests, platelet transfusion. Finally, at six in the morning, we were allowed to sleep. I was on a cot next to David's bed when the sun crashed in, awakening us with a start.

"Well, Mary, here we are. The first morning out of the bubble."

"Yes, our first sunrise."

"Wrong. We've shared lots of sunrises. We could see the sun come up through the den window at the house. But we couldn't touch it like this. You know there is one good thing about this."

I nodded as he laughingly stated, "Right, no cameras. The first historical event in the life of the Bubble Boy not captured on film."

"Mary, there's dust in here."

Knowing he equated dust with germs, I tried to reassure him that the room was sterile: "I'm gowned from head to toe."

"No, no. I see dust; the breeze is moving it. I feel it in my nose. Get off the cot and come look from here."

From his viewpoint I could see lint in the streams of sun coming through the mini-blinds. With relief, he accepted my explanation: lint from the sterile bed linens.

"Mary, look again. They're minute snowflakes."

I stood looking at him as he smiled and toyed with the sunbeams. He was so handsome, those black, expressive eyes so alive—no more leaden look. He needed a shave; strange, I had never noticed before.

Abruptly, the sun disappeared. David demanded, "What happened? Pull up the blind."

It couldn't be. Only a tiny patch of blue sky. It was too cruel. Wasn't it enough that he was dying?

"Mary, Mary, answer me. What is that?" "A brick wall."

"It's the solid brick wall in *The Monster at the End of This Book*. You hated the book, and now you hate the wall."

"It's all right. We're together. How did all this happen? What went wrong?"

"David, I don't know. The doctors are baffled. They don't even know if it's the transplant."

"No, no. Not the transplant. Not now. I mean when it all started."

Just then Jackie entered. "Hi, how did it go last night? Did you get any sleep?"

"Not much. It must be eight o'clock. I have to get dressed and go to my office."

"Okay, go, but I'm warning you—prepare yourself. We are going to finish this discussion. See ya."

David knew nothing of normal sitting; when told to sit up, he knelt and sat on his heels. Out of the bubble, assuming different body positions proved to be a harrowing experience for him. The nurses, trying to change the bed linens, had David sitting on the side of the bed, feet dangling. His father said, "I'll help." He put one arm under his son's knees, and the other around his back, and swiftly lifted him off the bed. David's scream of terror brought all of CRC to the anteroom. His father quickly set him back on the bed, and I rushed to hold him.

The first time David sat in the room's reclining chair, it was firmly shoved into the corner and did not tilt. The second time, we moved the chair parallel to the bed so he could watch TV. I warned, "Be careful. This chair tilts back like this."

He let out a blood-curdling scream and shouted, "You're making me fall!"

"I'm not making you fall. Leaning back makes it tilt." The nurse said that the chair had moved back five degrees; at most, David wanted to get back in bed, but I protested, "I'll hold the chair steady."

He couldn't relax and repeatedly asked, "Are you sure you're holding it? Don't dare move and let me fall!"

I asked Dr. Shearer, "How long do I stay sterile? My germs must work through when I'm in the same garb for hours."

He replied, "About twenty minutes. It's a charade we have to keep up."

I agreed. "David couldn't tolerate people in here if he didn't believe he was in a germ-free environment." I was afraid that I would catch a cold and then not be allowed in the room, but I didn't.

With David out of the bubble, his parents and I settled into the routine of alternating staying all night. I spent every possible minute with him during the day, never leaving until nine or ten o'clock, and arriving at dawn.

Dr. Feigin came early, late, and in between; we seldom conversed, but David enjoyed the quiet time of having the full attention of both "the big boss" and me. Dr. Shearer, in and out, day and night, discussed in detail what was to be done and why.

David reclined, half-sitting in bed like a potentate, and consulted on his case with high-ranking physicians and section heads. His dignity, keen mind, and presence commanded respect. In this horrific situation I proudly watched him use the coping skills I had taught him. In addition, he played an impressive role, one learned from his mother—always smile, always be polite, never complain, and never show a hint of anger. After completion of a painful procedure, he would thank the physician.

Thursday, the phone rang and rang. David startled at every ring and finally said, "That phone is driving me crazy! Every goddamn person in Conroe has my number. I need peace and quiet." Marla took the phone off the hook, and that's where it stayed.

Bill, as I expected, asked about David's view. When I told him there was nothing to see, he brusquely demanded, "What do you mean nothing? Surely he has a window"

"Yes he does, but a brick wall obstructs the view."

Bill gasped and after a long pause chokingly sputtered, "That is the saddest thing I ever heard—incredibly sad, bureaucracy at its finest. Mother, I've been wrong. Even you never stood a chance against it."

I replied, "Some ways, yes. Some ways, no. But complete failure—no."

Saturday night, the eleventh, so much went on, one procedure after another, and the needles in his arms plugged up. Finally, after midnight, David and I were by ourselves. I remarked, "It is nice with the hustle and bustle gone. Being alone is great."

"See Mary, everything is the same. I told you that nothing would change between us when I was out. Everything would be the same, nothing would ever change between us."

I had tried to maintain my composure, but this was too much for me. I buried my head in the pillow and sobbed.

The next day Dr. Shearer explained, "We are going to do a rectal biopsy to diagnose GVH disease. This is most unusual because GVH has a set pattern of clinical symptoms and is not diagnosed by biopsy." Dr. Kathleen Motile could not get a tissue sample so Dr. Shearer and I assisted. What a mess—blood, mucus, and feces, all over the plastic sheet.

I thought, "Thank goodness David can't see this," and asked, "If he had a bowel movement, would that help?" She said yes. Dr. Shearer, David, and I made the trek to the bathroom. With practice, we had gotten pretty good at this awkward chore. When David was back in bed, Dr. Motile succeeded.

After gathering her equipment, she hesitated leaving, "Do they leave you two alone?"

David replied, "All the time."

Dr. Shearer returned and asked, "Mary, do you know anyone with A positive blood? He'll probably need another transfusion."

"My nephew, and he's healthy." "Which one?" David interrupted. "Robby."

"He's the one that's got money. I won't have Robby's blood—absolutely not."

By now, the donor skin graft on David's arm was an inflamed blistery pox—like a huge, angry smallpox vaccination. He was given a local anesthetic on his upper left arm for a "punch" biopsy. Three small circles of skin were snipped out—one from the donor graft, one from the graft of David's own skin, and the third from between the two grafts. This procedure looked painful to me, but David told Dr. Moise Levy, "It didn't hurt. Thank you."

The pathologist, Dr. Mary Gresik, asked me to describe the skin grafts and the recent eruption. I asked what she was looking for in all the biopsies. She said, "I'm not sure—cell changes of any type." She continued to explain and invited me to come down to the laboratory to see the process. She was doing it by hand so she could have results in a few hours, instead of the normal twenty-four hours.

Near noon, Dr. Shearer asked, "Mary can you get your nephew in here?"

"Yes, he's waiting for a call. I have to get him, but it won't take long."

David pitched a fit again; he did not want Robby's blood, and he did not want me to leave.

I cautioned Robby, "Please don't tell anyone you're donating blood. A public announcement of how gravely ill he is will bring donors, but it will also bring the reporters and curious people." The blood bank, closed on Sunday, opened for Robby, and after a two-hour physical examination they took his blood.

Later, Dr. Shearer explained that the biopsy demonstrated cell changes presumed to be graft-versus-host disease and he was starting steroid treatment. He answered David's questions about giving monoclones with, "There's no point. You don't have any T-cells to clone out."

Monday, David asked, "Why doesn't Potts come in the room? Why does she stand outside the door to talk?"

I said, "She can't bear to see you so ill." He nodded. "Oh."

Potts and the rest of us were working hard to make David's stay outside the bubble as enjoyable as possible. She had finally found a sterile cola drink; but he could no longer swallow. She had also taped a red metallic heart and Cupid on his door. Someone had brought in his wall clock. I sterilized the stained glass football player that his friend, Andrew, had made for David, and that was one of his most prized possessions. I stuck it on the window. David screeched, "Damn you, Mary, you could have ruined it!"

"No, I couldn't. Betadine and alcohol won't hurt glass."

Before six o'clock on Tuesday morning, Martha phoned me at home. "Don't panic, David's all right, but we need more blood. Can you find donors?"

I said yes, but thought, it's not even daylight. Where am I going to find Type A blood donors who will keep their mouths shut? My brother and nephew had donated. Who cares enough about David and knows lots of people? The answer came: Tom Langford, David's "electrician" and longtime friend. He knows everyone in the medical center.

I phoned. "Tom, David needs blood, lots of blood. Please find some Type A positive and keep it quiet. We've got enough problems without having hoards of people descending on the hospital."

"Mary, it's done. How is he?"

"So terribly ill and going down fast."

I called Martha back, telling her that I had blood coming. I never for one second doubted Tom's word, and sure enough, by ten o'clock, the blood bank at St. Luke's Hospital had a long line of donors. Reports came back that many rejected donors broke down and wept.

Later that morning, Dr. Shearer explained that a triple catheter would be inserted in David's chest to facilitate transfusions, nutrition, and provide for quick medication. Around noon Carol Ann gave permission over the phone for the surgery.

When Dr. Robert S. Bloss implanted the subclavian line, there was no space for me in the room or the anteroom. Celine opened the door to assure me, "He knows you're here." For the first and only time during this ordeal, David screamed in pain. Martha and two others in the hall sobbed aloud. The roof of my mouth throbbed, went dry, and I felt as if I were being strangled.

Dr. Feigin came in and angrily accused, "You're maudlin!" My instant rage and the impulse to slap him was my first awareness of the extent of my terrible anger. I slumped back in my chair as he ranted on, "Why is everyone so upset? David is no different than any other patient! I have a hospital to run and there are a hundred children just as sick!" He walked out abruptly.

When he returned a short while later, I had calmed down and was able to confront him. "It's unfair accusing me of being maudlin. What do you expect? I come up here, Martha and others are crying. David is screaming. I can't go to him because of the space. He knows I'm here waiting. Further, I'm the only one not crying, and you won't ever see me cry."

He touched my shoulder. "There are other sick patients." "They're not mine."

As soon as one person came out, I went in. David held up both his arms and turned his hands in all directions. "Now, this I like. No needles. No tied-down hands."

Wednesday night, David and I were watching TV—waiting for his father who was going to spend the night. I complained, "That old TV rerun, we've seen it a dozen times. Let's find something else."

"You two must have known each other a long time," the nurse commented.

"How long?" David asked.

"Almost ten years," I said. "It's good to have a friend so long."

"No, I'm the lucky one. I had Mary ten years."

I reflected that it was the third time that day that I had heard him use the past tense to describe himself.

While David used a bedpan, a nurse tried to hold up a sheet as a screen. David ordered, "For heaven's sake, leave that sheet alone. It's just interfering."

She countered, "We must—someone's in the room." He impatiently ordered, "Drop that sheet. That's just Mary. She doesn't count." Despite other similar scenes, the ritual of my back being turned as he toileted continued. I prepared sterile washcloths, set the bedpan on the bed, and turned around.

Thursday morning, Dr. Shearer shook his head. "Mary, I don't know what to expect next. Every day it's a new crisis, something new, something unexpected. I don't know what's going on. All I can do is deal with each crisis."

I looked at David's grotesque body. It seemed as if all his flesh had moved to his stomach. His life had been an endless parade of little white washcloths in and out of the bubble. Now, his dying was an endless flow of blood—blood in and blood out of his body.

Weak though he was, he continued monitoring his own care. Once, he read 'O' on a bag of blood and demanded, "Get that out of here! I'm A positive. I will not have O blood."

Dr. Guerra said, "I'll take it back to the blood bank and talk with the doctor in charge." She returned and said, "O blood is universal and it's been irradiated." He ceased to object.

On February 16, I was leaning against the wall in the hall outside of David's room when Dr. Feigin put both hands on the wall over my shoulders and quietly told me, "It's mono from the transplant. It's the only explanation."

"Why wasn't it checked for?"

"You can't. There's no lab technique. The Epstein-Barr virus stays dormant and hidden in the cells."

"But Katherine hadn't been sick."

He said, "She probably had it a long time ago. Almost any donor would be carrying the mono virus—it's in more than ninety percent of the population. It probably will never be proven one hundred percent, but that's what it is. The virus has made what little immune system David had go berserk." Shocked beyond disbelief, my only thought was that we should not let David know that his sister's marrow was the source of his illness.

That day was David's worst day. It was also Carol Ann's birthday. Her parents and three sisters came from San Antonio to take her to lunch. Her father and I were sitting in the nurses' lounge when Carol Ann came in, climbed on his lap, and sobbed. As they left, her father asked me to call him if David's condition worsened. His grandmother wanted assurance that David was getting better. I couldn't answer either one of them; I just stood there.

David continued to deteriorate. On the twenty-first, David's grandfather said, "Last Thursday you told me my grandson was dying."

I countered, "I don't remember saying that."

"You didn't. Your eyes told me."

Father Connelly came to give David the sacraments for the very ill. Dr. Shearer would not allow the holy oil in the room and on David because of contamination and suggested a dry run with sterile water. Father Connelly refused; he had to use the holy oil.

The news releases became troublesome to Carol Ann. She said the family did not want any more bulletins about David's deteriorating condition. Public relations talked with her and insisted that they had to give releases. The public and the media demanded it.

That night, I felt as if I had lost David. We were never alone. Something was being done to him virtually every second, day and night—X-ray machines came in, special nurses, special monitors. From home, I called Louise, sobbing, "I've lost him. He doesn't need me. He has dozens of people working on him. There's no room for me."

Friday morning David whimpered, "Oh, Mary, I'm afraid I've been awfulizing."

"No, love, you're not awfulizing. Everything is awful except the way you're handling this. I'm proud of you. No one else in the world is as stoic and brave as you."

Saturday morning, February 18, David implored, "Please don't leave—when will you be back? It's Saturday, and Saturday evenings are mine. Come back this afternoon—please." I assured him I'd return after completing my mother's errands.

Mother and I stopped at my favorite dress shop, Ella Pryor's. Trying on a dress, I dissolved into tears. "David is dying, and I'm buying clothes. I have to get back."

Virginia, a saleslady and friend, tried to console me, and Mother said, "You have to have a break. How long can you go on thinking of nothing but that boy? Give yourself something. Buy that dress."

David Sr. called, wanting to know when I would be back. Mother declared fiercely, "You are not leaving until you eat a decent lunch!"

That evening Dr. Shearer, numb from fatigue, solemnly stated, "Son, you need rest. Mary, I'm going to leave you two alone tonight and let nature work."

Alone at last, we lay in silence. David sighed, "I wish we were home. I know what you'd be doing. You'd be eating a grapefruit. It's so stupid in here—no Fannin Street. Everything is stupid. You're stupid. Why don't you just go over there and lie down and go to sleep? Quit trying to talk. Quit interfering."

After a while, I said, "I need a drink and bathroom break. I'll be right back."

As I took off my gown he yelled through the intercom, "Mary, get back in here! Why so long? What are you doing?" Back with him, I said, "At your command, your majesty."

"Lay down! Go to sleep! Be quiet!" He muttered "Stupid, stupid," and savagely cursed. Deciding enough was enough, I stood up. He grabbed my outstretched hand.

"I'm in a box, in a prison. Where is the world? Oh, Mary, there's not one part of my body that doesn't hurt. I should have killed myself before. I should never have agreed to this." He cursed repeatedly. "Would my way last summer have been easier?"

"I don't know. I just don't know."

"Mary, it's all right. We'll never know. I should have died years ago, before I was old enough to care. Maybe I should never have been born. No, no that's not right. That was okay. It's what they did to me. They should never have put me in a cage and treated me like a wild animal. They didn't care about me. Even if they didn't care about me, didn't they know they were dealing with a human when they boxed me?"

He began more venomous curses, over and over. "Where are those three that did this to me? The ones that never thought about what they were doing to the life of a human being—my life. I haven't seen them around. Well, they wouldn't be around when we're up to here in shit. It's all their fault. They did this to me. The prison and now my arm—the graft—she did it all. The smartass bitch never cared. I was her claim to fame."

"David, I should have said come out last summer. I should have uncapped you, and we could have had a few good days."

"No, Mary, we don't know that. Why? Why? Why did this happen?

What happened? What went wrong?"

"We don't know. Nothing went according to plan. I didn't want this for you."

"I know. I mean from the beginning, not now. Why? Why? Is there any meaning to this? Is there any meaning to my life?"

"I don't know the meaning of life," I said. "I don't know the meaning of death. I don't understand why we live. I don't understand why we die. No one does."

"How can you and I know the answers? We don't know the questions. There has to be some meaning to my life. Why did I live? I need a reason. Give me a reason."

"There has to be a meaning. I don't know what it is at this moment. Your life could never be for nothing. I don't have the answers except the one for me. Your life has had more meaning for me than anything else. I love my son, but what you and I have is so different, so special, so precious. I bet few people have ever been friends like you and I."

"Oh, Mary, you will be lonely without me."

"Yes, my love, I will."

"Everyone should have a reason for having lived. Tell me there is and will be meaning to my life. You're right, there has to be meaning. Someday you'll know. Oh, Mary, where is the world? I never knew the world. Oh, Mary, where, where is it? I wanted the world."

"I wanted the world for you. More than anything I wanted it for you."
"It's all right. You tried. Mary, you were the world. I didn't know the world

and the world didn't know me. It should know me and everything that happened to me. You know. You tell the world. Promise."

"Love, I will. I promise."

"Mary, you know what your trouble is?"

"No."

"You care too much. You don't have enough sense not to care."

"Love, let me tell you—"

"Oh, Mary, shut up. I know exactly how you feel." Gripping my hand tighter and pulling me close, he sobbed loudly and convulsively. A nurse opened the door; I motioned her away. The regular CRC nurses felt relieved that he had at last cried.

After he went to sleep, I threw myself on the cot and sobbed. I refused to let myself doze off for fear someone might wake him up. If the door opened, I dashed over; "He's asleep. Don't talk or make noise. If you wake him up, I'll kill you."

After three hours, David awoke, serene, smiling, and softly repeating my name over and over. "Do you remember our two-story house—our real spaceship—our lovely messes? Remember the time you were really upset?"

I was at a loss about that last one. What about right now? Which of a hundred other times?

"Oh, you know, you were really upset; I mean really. I came back to the hospital with a new curse word, the N-word. You couldn't figure it out and thought I was teasing. When I spelled n-i-g-g-e-r you were shocked, stunned. Oh! Gee! Were you upset! You stood there with your mouth wide open a long time and finally said, 'Oh, David, that's a terrible word. You can't ever say it again. It's not a curse word.' "

"I argued—it is a curse word. I heard it on cable, and my father's friend called a football player that when he dropped the ball. You said, 'Listen, I don't care if you say the F-word, the B-word, but never, ever, ever can you say that word. It's not a curse word. It's a derogatory word. It offends me and violates my beliefs. My rule: never allow that word spoken. It humiliates black people'."

"I never, ever, said that word."

"I know you didn't. If you had, you would have been in big trouble with lots of people besides me."

"Remember how we played the 'N' game? Let's play it now. I say, guess what? I learned a new curse word, the N-word—now be horrified. This time could we please actually say the words?"

We played the game over and over, saying curse words, but never, ever the N-word. Smiling, he went back to sleep.

At dawn he opened his eyes, smiled, and reached out his hand. I told him, "I am going to lie down, but I am so tired I might go to sleep If you want or need something, just say it louder."

"Mary, Mary, I don't have to say it any louder. You always hear me. You wouldn't ever not hear me."

Sunday morning the physicians came in as usual. Again Dr. Shearer left us alone. Dorothy and a new young nurse, Ellen, were on duty. One of David's fluffy white boots that kept his feet warm and prevented friction burns on his heels fell off. As I struggled to get the straps fastened, he yelled, "Stupid! Stupid! Can't put a simple boot on!"

Ellen scolded, "Don't be so mean to Mary!" then cried and ran out. David stared at me a long time. "Oh, hell, I know it doesn't matter what I say or do—you will never leave me."

I thought, you're right, I'll never leave you. But you are leaving me. Dorothy came in and suggested, "Go eat. I'll stay awhile. Ellen is upset, talk to her."

"Dorothy told me not to worry," said Ellen, still crying, "You and David go back a long way, and you knew what you were doing. But it's not fair. He's so mean to you and you're so kind to him."

"It's all right," I said. "I'm tired of his verbal assaults, but he's so angry, in so much pain. He has a right to be angry, and it has to go someplace. He wouldn't dare direct anger toward anyone else. To tell you the truth, I couldn't stand apathy. Anyway, his anger is almost gone."

Sunday was a long, long day. Even with oxygen, David could hardly breathe. He would tire of the facemask so I took it off and held the oxygen hose at his nose. He complained of being smothered—no air –and boredom. When I suggested TV, he said, "Have you ever looked at a TV Guide for Sunday afternoon? What do you suppose is happening to Westheimer? Do you think it can hold together? Gosh, we haven't done anything about it lately. You'll have to get it straight when this is all over. You'll have time."

Dorothy came in, holding up a handful of markers. "This room is so barren, I had to do something. They're sterilized. You can draw on the sheet of paper from inside the glove packs." David smiled, reached for the markers, admired them from all angles, and caressed them. In a half-sitting position, he arranged and rearranged them on his chest and finally said, "We need something to put these in." We put them in a beaker from the medical cart and he went to sleep looking at them propped under his arm.

David's deterioration that day brought on more heroic measures. With a giant needle, Dr. Bloss extracted fluid from his chest cavity, allowing him to breathe easier. Dr. Shearer, expressing great reservations, placed him on acyclovir, an antiviral medication.

Carol Ann came around six o'clock. David was asleep. I told her I would stay all day Monday because it was President's Day. The next morning, Carol Ann, distraught, stated, "I cannot go in that room again. Last night was terrible. Dr. Shearer will not give me hope." I hurried to David.

Dr. Shearer came in, shook his head, and said, "Nothing went the way we planned. I don't know what's caused David's basic reaction here—an infection or B-cell neoplasm (cancer) from the transplant."

Specialists came in and out. I thought Dr. Shearer had ceased treatment, but Jackie said, "They will never give up as long as his mind is so clear."

The anteroom looked like something between a disaster area and a storehouse. Supplies were piled high on the cot. Everything got pushed against the walls to make room for the X-ray machine and other large equipment that was periodically brought in. Dr. Larry Jefferson, head of critical care, and I kept one little corner of the cot clear where we could half-lie or sit. I kept a stash of report-writing supplies under the cot.

My schedule at CDP continued to be full, but testing a child was a reprieve from misery and grief. I could take a child into the testing room and forget everything.

Monday night was an extension of the day. David grew weaker, dozed more, but remained cognizant of everything going on. My beautiful love—only his hair and his eyes remained beautiful. He wanted me to be looking right at his face when he awoke so that our eyes would lock.

Once, when my head nodded down, he opened his eyes and yelled, "Mary, pay attention to me!" For what seemed an endless time, David looked into my eyes. I didn't know what he was seeing. I don't know what I was seeing. What was he trying to find in my eyes? Was he looking for his own immortality? I had told him that love is always now and never dies. Was he seeing love? Was he looking into my eyes for comfort, or was this a way of holding onto life?

Very early in the morning, Dr. Feigin and I stood facing each other across David's bed. Sunbeams hit David's face as he smiled and gazed from Dr. Feigin to me and then dozed off. Dr. Feigin looked into my eyes with the same intensity as David had. But this was different. I felt Dr. Feigin's eyes see inside me. I wondered, what does he see? My pain? My exhaustion? My anguish? Then I had a strange but fleeting thought: if there is such a thing as a soul, and if I have one, he is seeing it.

Tuesday, Dr. Larry Jefferson took complete charge. Dr. Shearer's nurse, Lynn Papsy, formerly a critical care nurse, took charge of supplies and coordinated all activities.

Late that afternoon, after my last CDP appointment, I went into David's room. Larry, holding David's hand, said, "Open your eyes. Here's the hand you want to hold." David looked at me, smiled, and dozed off.

At about half past seven David was sound asleep and I told Larry, "I'm going home. I can't make it any more."

He said, "I have your phone number, but write it on the mirror in the anteroom."

I got as far as the door, turned around, and said, "Larry, I can't leave."

"Good."

Dr. Clayton had all the CRC patients, except the SCID infant, moved to other units. He thoughtfully put couches in the hall. As the relatives arrived, I would tell David. Many times he asked, "Who is out there?"

"Both sets of grandparents and all your aunts and uncles." He commented, "That's the way it should be."

I did not like talking with members of the extended family. With the exception of Carol Ann's father, none seemed to believe David was dying. They asked "Is he better? Don't you think he's better than he was?" They had no idea of what things were like with David, and I wasn't about to be the one to tell them.

Each time I came out of David's room, they reached out to me. One time Carol Ann's mother looked right at me and asked, "He's going to be all right?"

I said, "No. Your goals are different from mine. All I want for him is comfort, and you're still hoping for life." At one point it seemed like at least two dozen arms were reaching out to me, and I explained, "I'm sorry, I can't give any of you anything. All of my energy is down there in that room."

Carol Ann's mother said, "That's where we want it to be."

At nine o'clock that night, I was holding David's hand when Jackie came in. She said, "My husband told me to come back. He said my heart was here." I cried in relief and left the room for a while.

A few minutes before ten o'clock, David said, "Turn on the TV. I want to watch *Star Trek*." We turned the volume as loud as possible, but he still couldn't hear over all the machine noises. The TV itself had no knobs to turn. All of a sudden, getting the volume loud enough for him to hear was the most important thing in the whole world. I climbed up on the medical cart and used surgical instruments to poke inside the TV.

Jackie commented, "Who would believe he knew it was time for *Star Trek*? Who but you would be in that precarious position, adjusting the TV and actually getting it louder?"

While Larry worked with David, Jackie and I sat in the hall. David Sr. sat down and put an arm around each of us. "I want to thank you both for loving my son."

David wanted Jackie and me both to hold a hand, but at half past twelve, Jackie concluded, "This can go on for quite a few nights. We can't both stay all night every night. You stay tonight and I'll stay tomorrow night." She left and I continued to hold David's hand.

He awoke agitated.

"I'm crazy. I'm crazy. I don't understand all this. I'm losing my mind."
"No, you're not going crazy. You hurt. You're angry. You can't get well.

You have the right to feel angry, but you're not going crazy."

"Yes, I am. I am crazy, I know I'm going crazy."

"No, no, you're not going crazy. You are my love, and my love will never be crazy. I won't let you be crazy."

On and on, back and forth, until Dr. Fawcett, a fellow of Dr. Shearer's, interjected in a loud, jarring voice, "David, listen to her, she's right. You're not crazy."

After a pause, David questioned, "I'm not crazy?"

"Love, everything that has happened is crazy—this room is crazy, but you are not." He dozed off.

When he opened his eyes and I had my head turned, he yelled, "Mary, pay attention to me!"

"I am."

"No, you're not. If I open my eyes, I want to see your eyes." If I moved my hand, he woke up. He pleaded, "Turn the oxygen higher, I can't breathe. It's not on high."

At two o'clock, Larry told me he would be busy with David for at least thirty minutes. I said, "I'll go home to get a change of clothes."

David pleaded, "You'll be right back?"

I promised, "Half an hour at the most."

Around three o'clock, the blood pressure gauge read zero, and the beeps stopped. I thought, "He's dead—it's a peaceful moment." But Larry came running in, pumped something into the central line, and beep, beep—everything was going again. David opened his eyes and smiled.

One moment I wished for David to have peace and be free of pain, the next minute I petitioned, "Please let me have him one more minute." Because I simply could not stand up any longer, I knelt on a sheet on the floor, but it didn't work very well. It was uncomfortable holding my arm up to hold his hand. I put another sheet on the bed and sat on it.

Then I glanced up and saw a metal box break off the wall hook on which it had been hung. It seemed to take hours to fall. As it went down, I thought: I can't move. I must not move.

I didn't. The box crashed to the floor but David never stirred. Yet if I moved my hand even the slightest, his eyes would open.

There, with him sleeping, I knew that David now totally accepted death. The anger was gone, and there was not a hint of fear.

Early Wednesday morning, Drs. Shearer and Feigin came in. Dr. Shearer explained that David was to be given sedation and put on a respirator. Dr. Feigin told me, "You have to leave. There's no room for you in here."

I explained to David, "It's half past eight, and I have to present the first case at the case conference. I'll be back in an hour." Groggy, he seemed puzzled, and I repeated myself. Dr. Feigin, impatient at what he thought was my resistance to leaving, tugged at my arm. "No, wait, I'm trying to explain to David that I have to leave but will be back. David, if you want me before an hour, have Dr. Jefferson call. I'll drop everything and come back."

David murmured, "All right. Mary, remember I love you very much. Goodbye."

As I ran down the three flights of stairs to the case conference I thought something's different, something's wrong. After awhile it hit me—David never tells me goodbye. What does he say? I couldn't remember.

After the conference and back up at CDP, Mildred said, "A man—I think Dr. Shearer—called and wants you up on CRC."

The CRC hall was a freeway for medical equipment. Physicians ran in all directions. Dr. Jefferson said, "A few minutes after you left, David fell apart."

I cried, "Oh, no! His mind or his body?" "Body, Mary, body. Everything."

"I'm sorry I left, I should have stayed!"

"No, Mary, I'm glad you weren't there—you didn't need to see that. He had the sedation."

Jackie said, "I got here as you ran out—I was too late. He was unconscious."

I asked, "Jackie, what did David always say when I left?"

" 'See ya!' "

Jackie, Potts, and I were together when Potts heard the word "cancer." It was the last straw. She swooned, someone took her home. With two hands, Jackie pushed Dr. Feigin into a room.

"Is he dying?" she asked. "Yes."

Dr. Shearer repeatedly assured me that David was not conscious or suffering. "The last thing he might possibly remember is the priest at ten. I got the holy oil sterilized."

My stomach hurt so bad I had to call Mildred to find my pills. She brought me one. Later, I called her again. I was freezing and needed my jacket. This time, she held me in her arms for a long time while I cried.

Raphael Wilson came rushing in with Carol Ann, who said, "Dr. Feigin, I would like you to meet Dr. Wilson." Raphael reached toward me saying, "I've got to talk to you." Revolted, I cringed as he headed toward me with extended arms. He never approached me again. I knew a senseless, horrible anger was consuming me, but I didn't seem to be able to do anything about it or even care. I was sorting people into two piles—no in-betweens. Either I was angry with them or I wasn't.

At half past four that afternoon, Dr. Shearer came out and asked David's parents, "Do you want to go in? This will be the last time."

They both said no. Carol Ann looked at me pleadingly and I asked, "Do you want me to go in?"

"Would you please?" Jackie said, "I'll go, too."

We rushed to the anteroom and were gowning up when Dr. Shearer said, "I don't want you two to go in. It's too terrible. I don't want you to remember David this way."

Jackie and I went into a nearby room and clung to each other sobbing aloud. A nurse came in and said, "Hurry, gown up and get in David's room, Dr. Shearer wants you."

As several nurses helped us dress, Katherine came in and started to gown up. I asked, "Do your parents know you are going in?"

"He's my brother! I can do what I want! You can't stop me!"

"Katherine it's not that," I said. "You have every right to go in. It's just that this will be hard on you, and they should know that you're here."

Lynn Papsy, the nurse, explained the monitors—the beeps and flashes were residual electrical charges, not life, and would continue for quite awhile. She apparently thought it was important that I understand, because she repeated it. I thought, You don't have to hit me over the head with it; I understand.

Clean sheets and the Big Bird blanket covered David; all we saw was his right hand and face. I touched my forehead to his forehead. It was the first time my skin ever touched his. It was warm; it felt good. Jackie and I said our goodbyes, then clung to each other before going to David for one more goodbye. I kissed his cold hand and said, "Goodbye, my love."

Jackie said, "I love you—goodbye."

One of the doctors took me in his arms. Jackie and I walked out together.

The grandparents looked at us. I announced, "He's dead."

22.

THE FUNERAL

"He's dead," is all I could or wanted to say. Carol Ann's parents hugged me. As I went out the door, Jackie said Dr. Feigin wanted to see us both.

In his office, we all three cried. We sat on a couch, he in the middle with an arm around each of us. "Jackie, Mary, I want to tell you how much I appreciate your efforts and thank you for all you did. Thank you."

I cruelly rejected his attempts at consolation by dumping my regrets. "It's all my fault!" I sobbed. "I convinced him to go through with the transplant!"

"No, David wanted it," Dr. Feigin said softly. "It was what he wanted. Mary, Sunday night he knew he was dying—we discussed it."

"I know."

Suddenly I was nothing but tired; I wanted to be alone.

Jackie and I left his office. She headed back up to CRC; I went to my office to get my purse and then drove home. I called Mother, my cousin Anita, and dearest friends. After a hot bath in my whirlpool, I slumped into bed.

Tom Langford phoned. "I know. They called me to get ready for the press conference in the morning. Are you all right? Do you need anything?"

"No, thank you." I was oblivious to his own grief.

Jackie phoned near eight o'clock. "Both Carol Ann and Dr. Feigin asked me to call. Carol Ann is concerned because you're alone and haven't slept for so long. Dr. Feigin wants you to know they are going to pronounce the time of death as 8:00 p.m. He's afraid you might be upset if you hear the time on TV, since David was dead when you left."

I asked, "Why eight?"

"Possibly it's because he was on life support machines. David Sr. wanted to leave immediately, but Carol Ann objected and he stayed awhile. They are allowing Carol Ann's mother to be alone with David after the machines are out of the room. Carol Ann has agreed to an autopsy except for David's eyes."

In the morning, I awoke with my face on a sopping wet pillow. The intense sadness. I didn't know it was possible to cry while asleep.

Yet, despite the grief, I had another feeling—a burden was gone, no more despair about the future, David's or mine. I came to realize that I had no regrets, no feelings of guilt. David had absolved me from guilt. Without guilt, I somehow felt good about myself. My son and Lorna phoned, both crying. Bill's only concern was my wellbeing. Their houseguests and servants had cried with them when they heard of David's death.

The Rev. Raymond Lawrence called from New York to offer condolences. "I'm probably one of the few people outside of a small circle who realizes the magnitude of your loss. So few knew what this boy and you meant to each other," he said.

"Everything was perfect, so right, between David and me. I was with him all the time."

"I'm glad."

"No one interfered. Jackie was there, too. Every physician admired David and treated both of us with respect and compassion. He died with dignity, without fear."

I attempted to get out of bed, but my body was so heavy I plopped back down. Then, a momentary fantasy: I'll go to work and David will be at the window, waving. Uncontrollable sobs took over, but I decided that if I couldn't face this morning, if I couldn't drive into the parking lot this morning, I'd never be able to do it.

Wanting to talk with Barry about this inexplicable good feeling mixed with my grief gave the impetus to get me going. When I drove into the parking lot, the magical thinking returned: I'll look up and he'll be waving. He wasn't.

Carmen Dickerson, the only one in CDP, reached out to me. We embraced, both crying.

I rushed on to Barry's office, explained my feelings, and asked, "Why?" With tears in his eyes, he held me and said, "You know why, don't you?" "No. I don't."

"Because you were successful. You were successful in creating and maintaining an intimate relationship with another human being against all the obstacles in the world. Your relationship—your intimacy with David—was a divine gift of God, one that few people ever know."

Back in my office, one by one, my colleagues extended their condolences. Everyone in the clinic cried. I looked at the Thursday schedule. I had no appointments.

Immediate anger took over—why no kids today? But it was pointless anger: When they had made the schedule they hadn't known David would die yesterday.

Jackie called. "Let's meet on CRC and go through David's things. Carol Ann told me we could take whatever we wanted."

We opened the door to his room—the bubbles and playroom were gone. David's things were heaped in a pile and on top sat the green fuzzy frog. I grabbed it, buried my head in its tummy, and cried.

Jackie, crying, said, "I'll take the cowboy hat. What are we going to do if we can't stop crying?" I took the frog, the pumpkin, and a sketch of Fannin Street David had drawn in November. I looked for the Beatles record but the records and the player were gone.

Jackie said, "Big Bird is not here—we've got to find it." We went to the quarters where David had died—no Big Bird. We shuffled through everything, but no Big Bird. Jackie lamented, "It's gone to the laundry. We'll never get it back." I took Andrew's football player off the window and retrieved my stash of report-writing supplies from the anteroom. Jackie went off in search of Big Bird.

I went to Dr. Shearer's office. He stood up and walked toward me; we reached out to each other and locked into each other's arms, crying.

"Why did he have to suffer? Why did he have to die? It isn't fair."

Then I heard David say, "Oh, Mary, you won't believe—" Startled, I pushed back and realized Dr. Shearer was speaking. "The preliminary autopsy findings—it's a breakthrough for medicine, for lives. It's the link between immunology and cancer. It's the evolution of cancer captured in frozen time frames. It would take more than twenty years of research in a laboratory to replicate this."

Stunned, I walked to the window. Looking at Fannin Street, I said, "Oh, God, if just David could have known; it would have meant so much to him. Why couldn't we have known before? Saturday night he pleaded with me to give him a reason for having lived. He wanted his life to have meaning. He saw it as wasted—he never accomplished anything worthwhile. If just I could have told him."

Dr. Shearer further explained the rapid reproduction of B-cells into lymphoma. The immunoblastic sarcoma had secreted the immunoglobulins.

Remembering Dr. Feigin's statement about EBV and proof, I inquired, "The virus, the cancer, will you know what is host (David) or what is donor (Katherine)?"

"Yes, but it will take months to sort out and I'll need help."

At that moment his secretary announced a long distance call. He looked at me and then at the phone and then back to me. Seeing his quandary I said, 'Go ahead." As I left several fellows approached me and one said that David had had 280 ulcers in his digestive tract. I had worried about one.

I went to David's room and watched Fannin Street, as I had done hundreds of times. Jackie returned, having given up the search for Big Bird. Everyone was discussing either the funeral time or the ten o'clock press conference. Jackie confided, "I can't tolerate driving to Conroe with a bunch of people. You and I need time together."

Back in my office, I called David's home. A friend who knew nothing of the funeral plans answered. Moments later Carol Ann's father phoned. He pointed out that the funeral time was not set, and that it would be invitation only, with a limited number of people attending. Knowing full well that I was being irrational, I began a diatribe against the people I didn't want to be invited.

Carol Ann called shortly, "Please come stay with us. The rosary is at seven tomorrow evening and the funeral Saturday morning." With thanks, I declined the invitation to stay at her home. She tried to persuade me, "You shouldn't be alone."

Friday morning, Jackie and I had coffee with Potts. That afternoon a memorial service for David was held in the hospital chapel, but I opted not to go. Tired, I went home. Judy brought me dinner. I dressed for the rosary and waited for Jackie. We didn't talk during the slow drive in Friday evening traffic. We arrived just as the service started. Sergeant Beeman greeted and seated us.

Afterward, Carol Ann's mother told us, "Big David is adamant that the casket remain closed, but after all the people are gone, it is going to be opened. I thought you two would want to see him."

We walked up to the casket. David, so peaceful, handsome, and grown-up, wore a blue velour shirt. There, in his hands, was his Big Bird blanket. Jackie whispered, "His grandmother must have done that." Jackie and I kissed him good-bye.

We declined Carol Ann's invitation to go to the house for a buffet, but agreed to attend the private service at the funeral home before David was taken to Sacred Heart Catholic Church for the mass.

Saturday morning, the day of the funeral, the sun was shining. It was a beautiful, warm day. Jackie and I alternated between crying and laughing on the drive to Conroe. Jackie had been right. We needed private time.

At the funeral home, Carol Ann said, I'm worried about my husband; he's blaming himself." I tried to speak with David Sr., but his sister, misinterpreting, told me this was not the time to bother him and pushed me away.

Drs. Shearer and Feigin, both obviously ill at ease, were standing in the anteroom. They didn't know the extended families or intimate friends. Jackie said, "Come on. They need us."

As we headed toward them, Carol Ann said, "Make certain Drs. Feigin and Shearer come to the house after the services. We have a buffet, and I'm sure they'll want to talk with the other doctors." I knew she meant the three original doctors. We three greeted Drs. Feigin and Shearer. Carol Ann invited them to the house but didn't mention "the other doctors."

David's friend Shawn, so grown up in a suit, came and embraced me. Ben, Raymond, and all the family friends came to me and expressed their thanks and sorrow.

Standing in silence next to Dr. Feigin, I recalled David directing my grooming and clothes at the time of the transplant. Would he think I was dressed all right now? My black and brown striped dress has a high neck, no buttons to gap. I turned to Dr. Feigin, "Do I look all right?"

"Why think about anything like that now? What difference does it make?" I didn't reply. Why try to explain? After the private service, we drove to the church.

The four of us followed the family into the church and sat behind David Sr., Carol Ann, and Katherine. The coffin was in the center aisle of the semicircle of pews, next to us. David's godparents, Dr. Bealmear and Raphael Wilson, sat on my left, Jackie was to my right, then Dr. Feigin and Dr. Shearer on the aisle. I glanced around. The church was packed and most faces were familiar. They sang my favorite hymn, "I come to the garden alone while the dew is still on the roses…" The sadness was overwhelming beyond words.

Father Connelly praised David's courage and made beautiful points about love. Then he droned on and on and on, comparing David's restricted life to that of his Down syndrome sister. After repeated references to "retarded," Jackie whispered, "If he says 'retarded' one more time I'm going to puke."

"David might yell 'Shut up!'" I said.

Dr. Shearer, a devout Catholic, followed the ceremonial rituals, and while he took Communion, Jackie and Dr. Feigin broke down. I turned to them, Jackie buried her head on my shoulder, and I put my left arm around her chest. Dr. Feigin reached for my right hand behind Jackie's back. We remained huddled together until Dr. Shearer returned.

When we filed out of the church behind the casket and family, we faced hundreds of people. We heard weeping as they stood motionless and silent. Dozens of photographers were on a knoll across the street.

Jackie and I were in awe of the miles-long crowd of sobbing, respectful mourners that we passed as the funeral procession wound toward the cemetery. The reporters and photographers who preceded the funeral procession stood around the edge of the cemetery. We could see telescopic lens cameras.

Under a tent at the gravesite, the four of us stood close together behind the seated family. Dr. Feigin comforted Jackie as she cried aloud when the six firemen played taps. I gasped, ready to sob, but Dr. Shearer gripped my arm and bid, "Now, Mary."

After the graveside service, Drs. Feigin and Shearer followed Jackie and me to David's parents' house. On the drive, Jackie said, "One time I almost laughed out loud. I looked around, all those cameras, hundreds of faces looking at us. I thought, they don't know you and me. They must think you're Mrs. Shearer and I'm Mrs. Feigin."

The four of us entered the house together but then parted. Jackie and I moved through the house and into the backyard because we couldn't bear the sight of the tables of food now sitting in the living-dining room area where the bubbles and playroom had been.

All the nurses, past and present, gathered around us. Carol Ann's sisters and their husbands thanked me for staying with David. After people had cleared away, I went into the living room. Carol Ann's father followed and held me for a long time. He never mentioned my bitter tirade over the funeral invitations.

On the drive back to Houston, we alternated between laughing, crying, and remembering. Jackie said, "Remember the time Dr. Desmond stuffed cinnamon buns down us so we wouldn't be tempted by Carol Ann's goodies?" It turned out we were both angry with the same people and incidents: David not being allowed to go into the parking lot, the parties where David was forgotten. Strange, we had never discussed any of this before. Probably we had never had time for chitchat.

23.

AFTERMATH

Monday morning after the funeral, I awoke crying. The music playing on my clock radio intensified my melancholy. The car radio, tuned to the same station, agitated me. I could not and would not listen to music for months.

I had been especially careful in applying my makeup and selecting my attire to assure that no one could say I wasn't handling my grief well. Dr. Frank Greenberg, a dear friend whose office adjoined mine, affectionately greeted me.

"I'm sorry I wasn't here for you last week," he said. "People in Philadelphia kept asking me questions about David. I didn't want to talk about him—all I could think of was you."

"Thank you for caring."

"A friend just back from Russia said everyone in Moscow cried at the news."

"Bill said, 'The whole world is crying.' "

"Do you realize your grief will be great and difficult to handle? You should channel it into something constructive."

Each day Frank continued to be a source of comfort. I didn't mind his knowing my distress. To everyone else at work I was, as Judy said, "composed and business as usual."

I deeply appreciated a phone call from Dr. Dean McDaniel, my dentist. "I'm very concerned because so few people know of your loss. When my son died during the holidays, the cards and sympathy of friends and acquaintances meant so much to my wife and me. You won't have any of that because no one knows."

He was right. Kaylen Fry, retired from Baylor Public Relations, wrote a letter of condolence. No one else except my close friends acknowledged my loss.

Potts came to my office with a brown box. "Here are all of David's favorite foods. I thought sometime when you were alone you would enjoy these and think of David." Although I was touched by her thoughtfulness, the idea didn't appeal to me. But she was right—I enjoyed eating the food, the chocolate pudding first, the tuna last.

I wrote Dr. Shearer a brief note in which I thanked him for allowing David to maintain dignity and control.

I concluded, "For a short time, you entered our private world and for that I will always be grateful."

More was involved in composing a letter to Dr. Feigin. We had been friends a long time, and I wanted to make amends for my behavior the evening David died. I wrote:

"Over the years, I've always felt your support and appreciation. You, more than anyone, seemed to understand the relationship between David and me. Thank you for always allowing him dignity. The one thing he and I most feared, the mind going before the body, never happened because of you.

"All of this was an ordeal for you, both personally and professionally. I am proud to be a member of your department and to know you. Ten years is a long time and I did not know it was possible to be so sad; yet, I have no regrets."

Dr. Feigin approached as I handed the note to Carrel Briley, his secretary, and asked, "Do you mind if I read this while you're here?" He did so, and with tears in his eyes, he murmured, "Thank you."

The next Sunday, Carol Ann and I attended Mass. Father Connelly invited us to his office to chat. He was elated over the publicity and requests for copies of his homily. Several people had advised him to write a book.

He remarked to me, "David was always so very polite, more than most boys. Did you see his polite behavior as being feminine?"

"No, that is ridiculous. David was the most masculine boy I ever knew. The politeness was his mother's influence."

The David Center was established at the hospital for the treatment and study of immune-deficient children. Carol Ann came to the hospital almost every day to answer the mail and write thank-you letters for the donations made in David's memory. She asked how I was handling my mail. When I said I had none, she told me, "The mail is yours as much as mine."

The outpouring of letters and donations prompted the hospital development office to suggest a book—a collaboration between the family, hospital, and a ghostwriter. The royalties would go to the David Center.

After a meeting with the parents, Drs. Feigin and Shearer, the development people, and Father Connelly, Carol Ann came to my office. She was "mortified." The joint venture ended when Father Connelly objected, "No Jew can write this Catholic story."

She left and Dr. Feigin came in my office and closed the door. I started to laugh and said, "Carol Ann just told me." He sat down saying, "I thought this Mickey Herskowitz guy was Polish."

Carol Ann decided to write an article for *People* magazine with Kent Demaret. He asked for my help and later wrote a thank-you note with the returned "material" which was a "great help during the structure of the two articles that challenged the icon of Happy Bubble Boy and presented David as a flesh and blood human being."

In *Newsweek,* March 26, 1984, Allan J. Hamilton writes: "The bizarre life and recent death of David, the boy in the bubble, have left me strangely upset. I am a physician and researcher, and David's story seems to pose serious and fundamental questions about human existence in general.... One cannot ask David or his family if living inside a bubble for 12 years was worth it.... We in research and medical communities must ask that question of ourselves.... The nagging doubt that I have about David was that he was never offered the option of volunteering to be part of the experiment, he was born into it."

In the *Journal of the American Medical Association,* January 4, 1985, the Rev. Dr. Raymond J. Lawrence, who had convened the 1975 ethics conference at St. Luke's/TCH, comments that with the exception of Hamilton's editorial, "I am not aware that any of the media has broached or even hinted at the profound and disturbing ethical and humanitarian issues that David's life raises.... David's life demonstrates the lack of attention in the medical establishment to the complex but critical question of what make human life human.... Our technology has run ahead of our philosophy, our religion, our value making and our ability to formulate the essential ingredients of the human."

He asked that the humanities, physicians, and scientists "explore and clarify the acceptable boundaries of the human."

Dr. Russell J. Blattner told me of his visit with Dr. J. Graham Watson in England. I said that Graham advised me to write a book about the "balmy people" around David.

Dr. Blattner laughed, "They were some strange ones. I have no idea where Dr. Wilson is now. He was a strange one."

"I thought of him as a mad scientist—sorta unctuous."

"That describes Raphael. Mary Ann was a strange one—the fundamental religion and rigid ideas. I was out of the city when it all happened, I made certain. I stayed out of it, left it to the experts. I knew it would be a tragedy. I was hoping that fellow (Shearer) who came later could do something. The transplant didn't work—a tragedy. His mother finally gets to hold him in her arms and he dies."

My day-to-day life went on. April 7, 1984, six weeks after David's death, Bill phoned.

"You're a grandmother. Laura Marie doesn't look like I expected. She has white fuzz for hair and blue-gray eyes, and she's twice as big as any of the other babies."

I laughed. "You expected a miniature Lorna."

He said, "Maybe. Right after she came out, the doctor dumped her in my arms, and asked me to check for myself that she was perfect. I had told him 'no heroic measures' if the baby was severely damaged. Mother, I've been around you too long." It was wonderful news, but my elation at having a granddaughter didn't take away from my sadness.

Each time Carol Ann and I went to Mass, we planned to visit David's grave, but invariably she decided against going. On April 14, 1984, family friends gave Katherine a Sweet Sixteen birthday party. Sergeant and Mrs. Beeman and I attended the outdoor festivity. For a few hours our mourning ceased.

Louise described me as "wearing blinders, charging straight ahead, writing the perception paper as a memorial to David."

Barry repeatedly told me, "You're wasting your time. You selected the most controversial issue imaginable. No matter which journal you submit to or how you write it, it will be rejected." It appeared that he was correct. I asked Jackie to be co-author. The first rejection was frustrating. The paper was lousy, but having the reviewers question the veracity of our observations devastated me.

I rewrote and submitted to another journal. In the middle of July, the editors notified us that, with revisions, they would consider publication. I worked at night to complete the revisions before Mother and I left for Singapore, the last day of August. Friday evening when I finally got on the plane, I was completely exhausted.

The plane landed at Taipei at sunrise. Everyone except Mother departed the plane while it was being serviced for the flight on to Singapore. Dozens of people from the plane entered the airport and disappeared. I walked up a flight of stairs to a long, long corridor, obviously a museum commemorating Chiang Kai-shek. Photographs and his portrait on huge stamps as well as exquisite paintings lined the walls. I decided to walk for twelve minutes and then turn back.

Time up, I stopped. The corridor seemed endless in both directions. A dreadfully eerie feeling enveloped me. I'm totally alone in this universe, alone in a cold tomb. No one could hear me scream. How is it possible to be so alone? I remembered David relating a dream of no one hearing his loud cries. Shivering and panic-stricken, I ran back to the plane.

Very few people had boarded so I moved away from Mother and burst into tears, thinking that surely this would be the last time for crying over David.

I forced myself to remember the happiest time yet since David's death. It had been an evening in March; I had gone for a walk at sunset, right after a shower. The new leaves, a delicate green, shimmered with raindrops. I looked at them awestruck, amazed to be reminded that there was still beauty in the world. Then suddenly, David was walking beside me. I did not see him, but felt his presence powerfully and heard his voice.

"See, Mary, raindrops are really diamonds. I know you are lonely without me, but don't be so sad. I'll always take care of you. I made sure." Then he was gone.

Eased by this memory, I soon fell asleep.

The flowers along the freeway were beautiful but Singapore as a whole was crowded—too many people, cars, and buildings. A magnificent garden with blooming orchids surrounded Bill and Lorna's luxurious home.

Within five minutes, Laura Marie's responsiveness and alertness told me she was precocious. She resembled her beautiful mother. But she was also Bill as an infant, and thirty-nine years evaporated in an instant as I watched her. Playing with her was pure happiness.

Surrounded by luxury, happiness, and love, I had another siege of sobbing. I realized that I could not replace one child with another. I had the most adorable, exquisite granddaughter in the world—somehow she should have taken away my sadness. But again, there was the thought, if I could just describe Laura Marie to David....

Later, when I told Carol Ann of this experience, she said, "I'm glad. I don't want another child to ever take my son's place in your heart."

Not enthusiastic over returning to work, I gave serious thought to resigning but everything changed the first day back. Everyone, including Dr. Feigin, welcomed me. "It's good to have you back," he said. "Are you all right? I've been worried. You were so far away the day you left."

"I was a sad sack—the paper and everything. We've not discussed our grief since the evening David died. I guess I, or we, couldn't. I wasn't prepared for the intensity of my sadness and anger. I miss him so much. He was mine."

"I know that."

"I never thanked you in person for your support. You helped me so much."

"No, you were the one that helped me," he said. "It wasn't easy for me, either."

"I know you cared for him and you also bore the ultimate responsibility." "You're great. One more thing, I will not allow you to get upset over that perception paper one more time. It's a beautiful paper and I thank you for writing it."

With my energy renewed, work didn't seem so tedious. The paper was rejected again. I revised it once more and submitted it to another journal. Life was easing. I went on shopping sprees and started an exercise program. My anger and grief seemed to be subsiding.

But it was not to be so simple. The night of December 4, 1984, I felt like hell. A haunting sadness overwhelmed me; once again, I had thought I was past this. Then, the grim realization: tomorrow is my birthday.

For years, David and I had celebrated my birthday together; for him it was a very special day. I relived my last birthday—David's "Surprise!" and efforts to be cheerful, my premonition of his death. And I remembered when he had asked me, "Why isn't your birthday picture in the newspaper, like mine?"

The next morning, the same feeling of dread. At work, it was banners, cards and ribbons on my door, and presents. Judy brought a tray of brownies.

I remarked, "You did this last year."

She replied, "I never told you this, but last year your birthday was on Monday. On Sunday, Andrew and I visited David, and he tactfully reminded me of your birthday—he didn't think I would want to forget. On the way home, we bought brownie mix. She and others announced, "We are taking you to lunch."

Shortly before noon Louise came in saying, "Come on, let's go to lunch. I want you to know that little guy up there is watching over you. This morning I woke up thinking of David. Believe me, I don't usually do that. I kept on thinking of him, and then I remembered it's Mary's birthday, so here I am."

At that moment Carol Ann, looking lovely and carrying a package with flowers, walked in. "My son would have expected me to remember your birthday. I made a special trip into Houston, just like last year when David insisted he had to have your present before seven o'clock."

Louise said, "I told her he's taking care of her."

I unwrapped the present—a beautiful red blouse. I saw Frank Greenberg walking down the hall with outreached arms. He held me. All my friends circled around us. I asked, "Frank, how did you know?"

"I just knew you needed my arms." Off to lunch we went and had a good time—no sadness. That afternoon Dr. Feigin, obviously glad to see me smiling, complimented me on my appearance. I told him about Carol Ann's arrival.

"I'm pleased with Carol Ann's thoughtfulness and your attitude, Mary. Last winter I watched you day after day after day with David. You were beautiful. I didn't know any person could be so beautiful. Did you know that all of my conversations with David concerned you? All he wanted to talk about was you. He worried about your being alone without him."

"I know. He thought I should marry."

"Why aren't you married? You should have a nice husband."

"You sound like a replay of David. Who should I marry? Do you have a man in mind?"

"Any one of the dozen in your life, or I'll find you a husband. Quit laughing. I'm serious."

"Too bad you're not older and single."

He, too, laughed, "Older—why?" and again expressed pleasure at my happy mood.

Alone in my office, I was surrounded by David's presence, and I heard, "Mary, were you surprised? Did you really like your birthday?"

"Yes, David, you made it a beautiful day." I smiled, remembering the delight in his eyes and the many ways he had expressed his love. I am the lucky one, I thought.

After work, I stood in the parking lot looking at Fannin Street. Then I walked backwards in order to see David's window. "My love," I said, "I'm glad I chose to love you." As I drove away, I listened to music on the car radio.

The next week the perception paper was accepted for publication in the *Journal of Developmental and Behavioral Pediatrics*. At the editor's suggestion, we put our intimacy with David "up front."

Jackie took over the revisions and correspondence.

She retitled the paper "Looking Out of the Bubble: David's Perception of the World." She also wrote an eloquent letter to the editor:

Although David's circumstances were unique, advances in modern science have confronted us with many children whose lives are altered as a result of dependency on medical technology. David's ability to explore the world was severely limited. The parallels between his irritations and those experienced by, for instance, children surviving attached to ventilators, are impossible to ignore. If our observations about David stimulate interest or even controversy about the way in which children in limiting environments grow and develop, then a closer look at these children would be a most fitting tribute to a very special and much-loved child.

February was a difficult month, marked by the death of a good friend. Jackie and Potts were sad and teary, discussing the upcoming anniversary of David's death. Potts decided the way to handle the anniversary of David's death (which she, Jackie, and I considered to be Monday, February 20, not Wednesday, February 22), was to stay at home.

In the meantime, the CRC staff had planned a surprise thirtieth anniversary party for Potts. I pointed out that she might not show up on Wednesday, the planned date. On Friday, the fifteenth, Jackie and I drove to Conroe to go with Carol Ann to David's grave. I wanted pinwheels for the grave, but couldn't find any, so I took white roses.

To my surprise, the ground was covered with sweet gum cones. I looked up. David's grave was under a tree. Nearby was the tallest tree I had ever seen. Jackie said, "Who would ever have believed we would miss the little toot so much."

Monday was President's Day. The upcoming CRC celebration on Wednesday seemed like the last straw. Tuesday was hell. Exhausted from the lack of sleep and confused, I couldn't separate the past from the present. I mixed up people and my feelings. I couldn't think or walk straight. I went into my office and sat, listless, drained, at my desk.

Late that afternoon, Dr. Feigin came to my office. My deterioration was obvious. He said, "Mary, you can't do this. I won't let you. I promised David I would take care of you. He made me promise I'd look after you."

I thought of David's "appearance" to me during my sunset walk. David had, indeed, made sure that I would be taken care of. I suddenly understood why Dr. Feigin had been hovering over me all through the year.

I went up to David's room. Dorothy Johnson came in. I told her what had just happened. Not at all surprised, she said, "As close as you two were, he would try to take care of you after he was gone. What better way than Dr. Feigin? You should write that book, Mary. It's David's legacy."

Late on Friday afternoon, February 22, the actual anniversary of David's death, I drove to Conroe in the rain to attend an evening memorial service at the Sacred Heart Catholic Church. As soon as I arrived, Carol Ann said the two of us needed private time with David even though the family planned to stop at the grave on the way to the service.

Carol Ann's voice startled me and brought me back to the present. "Mary, we must go—the memorial service, we've been here too long. They will be waiting for us at the house."

At the service, the young, handsome priest, whose face resembled paintings of Jesus, spoke from the Gospel of St. Mark. He said that from speaking with David's family and friends, he knew that David, like young Jesus, lost from his parents at the temple, had reached the age of wisdom. I felt a new sense of peace and wished this had been the homily at the funeral. After the service, which was attended by only a few intimate friends, I spent the night with David's family.

Saturday, after returning home, I collapsed with flu-like symptoms. Although I worked every day, I continued to have laryngitis for three weeks. My mental and physical collapse was probably long overdue.

On February 25, 1985, I was notified that I would receive the Myrtle Wreath, the highest honor conferred by Hadassah, the American Jewish Women's Organization. I was named, along with Jackie and Drs. Feigin, Shearer, and Desmond, for the prestigious award for distinguished medical and human service.

I had to get myself put back together before the awards dinner on April 20, so I followed Dr. Obenour's advice and started swimming at The Methodist Hospital Health Club at seven each morning. The swimming and an evening walk straightened out my sleep cycle and I was then able to function effectively.

On April 5, Dr. Shearer wanted to meet with me to discuss the final findings of the autopsy. When we met, it was as if the fourteen months since David's death didn't exist. We reached out toward each other, our grief just as acute as the morning after he had died.

Anguished, Dr. Shearer said, "Mary, I don't want to have to tell you this."

I said, "What is there to tell? Dr. Feigin told me it was Epstein-Barr virus and you told me you had evidence of the link between cancer and immunology."

"We sacrificed a human life. It isn't fair. This knowledge should have been learned without David's suffering and dying. It isn't fair to Katherine—an innocent, pure girl to carry such a burden. How can I tell the public her cells carried the lethal virus?

"I didn't want it to happen the way it did. I worry about Katherine, too. No child should donate bone marrow to two brothers and then have them both die."

"Why did T.J. thrive and David...?" He continued on with regrets about what he had and had not done, and about "sacrifice."

"Stop, stop. You're wrong. Don't think in terms of sacrifice—that's like deliberate, for science. David wasn't our experiment. He was angry with South and Wilson, not us. David was grateful for a dignified way out of an intolerable situation. You made the right, the only possible, decisions. Don't blame yourself. The possible alternatives to the transplant could have made horrible headlines. Don't you see, you gave him the one thing he wanted—his life not to be a waste. I'm fortunate. He made certain I had no guilt or regrets. I'm lucky I was able to keep my two promises—to be with him every step, and not let him lose control." It was a time of catharsis for us both.

Dr. Frank Greenberg escorted me to the Myrtle Wreath awards dinner. Jackie and I both received compliments on our elegant appearance. As Jackie, Dr. Shearer, Dr. Feigin, and I walked down a hall to have photographs taken, Dr. Shearer and I held hands.

Jackie whispered, "What's this hand holding?"

I smiled. "We worked through our grief together—we understand each other." She shook her head and laughed. Dr. Shearer gave the acceptance speech.

...It is difficult to place a value on any one person's life, but it is safe to say that the great teachers of history are long remembered and revered. David has taught us many things, not the least of which is courage, for he faced a life unlike any other human being's in history. The sight of that plucky youngster scampering through the portholes of the interconnecting parts of his isolator was an inspiration to millions of television watchers, burdened with their own special problems....

David died in his attempt to gain immunity but he has left us powerful lessons for the present and future. When the final studies of David's death are made and understood, I believe that David's life will be even longer remembered because of the new understanding of the importance of immunity in preventing infection and cancer. Viewed in that perspective, David's life was one of the most important in recent memory. It may be responsible for the prevention and the cure of diseases far more common than the one he struggled against....

...In all of nature there is the endless cycle of birth and death. So, too, with David, from the withered vines of apparent defeat have sprung up the tendrils of a new condition. From all over the world have come the good wishes, prayers, and support to establish The David Center at Texas Children's Hospital.

The confirmation of the link between Epstein Barr Virus and cancer was to be published in the May 1985 issue of *The New England Journal of Medicine*.

On September 17, Carol Ann invited me to dinner on the coming Saturday, David's fourteenth birthday. Two days later, Dr. Shearer told me he had asked Carol Ann to talk with the parents of a gravely ill child who was to receive a bone marrow transplant. He was not hopeful for the child's outcome. On Friday, September 20, Carol Ann came to my office after talking with the child's parents. She had dreaded coming to the hospital the day before David's birthday, but was glad she had. "It was good to see all the people on CRC."

Potts gave me money for balloons for David's grave. I found four perfect pinwheels, metallic silver with colored backs—red, blue, yellow, and green. Near my home, I sighted a new florist shop with pretty balloons floating around. I requested colorful balloons for a boy's birthday.

When the florist brought out one with "Happy Birthday," I said, "That's really not right."

"How old is the boy?"

I started to say fourteen, but then said twelve. I asked him to select plain, brightly colored ones.

"Lady, if you don't mind spending more money, I have one I think you would like." He brought out a beautiful big heart, one side silver, and the other red. He stuffed the balloons in my Mustang and closed the door. On the freeway, stuck in a traffic jam, I remembered the many trips to Conroe.

It was a beautiful day. As we drove to the cemetery, Carol Ann expressed her pleasure that I was writing a book. I reminded her, "The book may not be to your liking. The David I knew was not the David you knew."

She replied, "My son was special because he made the people important to him believe they were the most special one in his life. What you are writing will be the truth for you, but not necessarily the truth for how he was with me or with others." I agreed.

At the grave, I was busy with the pinwheels and balloons. The pinwheels, marvelous, twirled and twirled. A strong gust of wind blew the big heart off its stick. The balloon went faster and higher. Running with my arms up in the air in a futile attempt to retrieve it, I heard David laughing and calling, "Stupid Mary, trying to catch that balloon."

I sat down and Carol Ann, believing I was distressed, came running after me. I laughed out loud. "I just heard David say 'Stupid Mary!'" She smiled and we watched the balloon go high and get caught in the tall, tall tree.

I repeated the words spoken by David at age seven when we saw a pretty hot air balloon go by: "It's high, high in the sky... as high as a tree."

THE END

ACKNOWLEDGMENTS

I want to thank all those many unnamed persons who encouraged me to produce this book, and finally to place in public circulation Mary Ada Murphy's own account of the story of David Vetter before all the remaining principal players and witnesses are dead.

Others of whom I am aware have made efforts to disclose this story in whole or in part, but have not successfully reached the broader public. In part, to be sure, a large part of the public simply does not want to know. Among those known to me who have advocated a full disclosure of the Vetter story are the ethicists James W. Jones and Barron Lerner, as well as Barak Goodman and John Maggie in their *American Experience* television production, "The Boy in the Bubble." The late David McVickers of the *Houston Press*, published a candid report on the case. My friends Derrick Sherwood and Shannon Waltrip Sequeira have been energetically lobbying for full disclosure of the story.

I must give very high praise to Shannon Waltrip Sequeira who in proofing the first draft found a great many problems and errors with the proofs. Shannon is a very unusual person in relation to the David Vetter case. She herself is a close contemporary of David, just two years older. When she was eight years old she took a special interest in David's story. After his death she had personal communications with Mary Murphy. She is now something of an expert on the life of David Vetter. Shannon had much to do with motivating me not to further delay publication of this text.

I want to thank Jackie Vogel, Mary Murphy's colleague and friend, for her assistance in clarifying some of the details in the text that would be known only by someone who worked with David.

I am very grateful to all those who assisted me or spurred me on to put this book into the public arena, or who have done most of the work of getting this document into book form, especially Krista Argiropolis, David Roth, Derek Sherwood, Perry Miller, Cynthia Olson, Peter Roth and Howard Pendley.

And a special thanks to Charles Hicks, Esq., and his legal team at Health Law Associates in Little Rock.

I alone am responsible for any errors in the text.

For those who wish to see an extensive collection of photographs of David Vetter and his environment, the best source known to me is Houston's Baylor College of Medicine Library and its archive, which can be accessed through the Internet.

I am also happy now to be relieved of the burden I have carried around now for a quarter century, the burden of my promise to Mary Murphy to get her story into the public arena. With this publication I am grateful to have lived long enough to see my promise to her fulfilled.

ABOUT THE AUTHOR

Mary Ada Murphy

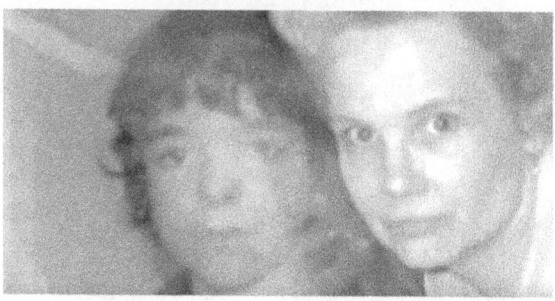

Born on December 5, 1926, Murphy first studied mechanical engineering and worked for many years as a quality control engineer in the Texas oil industry. In 1969 she earned a M.A. in psychology at University of Houston, and in 1980 received her Ph.D. in behavioral science at the University of Texas School of Public Health. Her dissertation was a study of the "Impact of Children with Birth Defects on Stress in Their Families." She was licensed as a Psychological Associate by the Texas State Board of Examiners of Psychologists, was appointed Instructor in Pediatrics at Baylor College of Medicine in 1970, and in 1982 was made Assistant Professor in Pediatrics.

Murphy was a Psychological Associate at the Meyer Center for Developmental Pediatrics at Texas Children's Hospital from 1969 to 1995, a Medical Staff Affiliate from 1984 to 1995, and a Member of the Pediatric Cardiac Transplant Team at Texas Children's Hospital from 1985 to 1995. From 1992 to 1995 she was a Medical Staff Person in Pediatrics for the Harris County Hospital District.

Murphy received the Hadassah Myrtle Wreath Award in 1985 in recognition of her outstanding achievement in the psychological support of David Vetter and his family.

She published nine papers and abstracts in various medical journals, most notably "Looking Out from the Isolator: David's Perception of the World" in the *Journal of Developmental and Behavioral Pediatrics*, Vol 6, No 3, June, 1985, with Jacqueline B. Vogel.

In 1995, Mary retired at age 69. She developed Alzheimer's and died in August 2013 at the age of 87.

ABOUT THE EDITOR

Raymond J. Lawrence

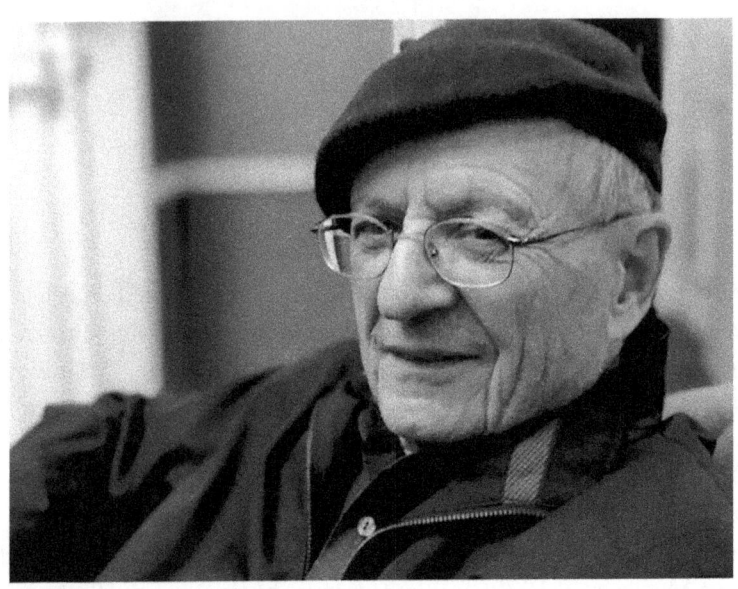

Raymond J. Lawrence is a Virginian by birth, who began his working life as a newspaper boy, then batboy for a professional baseball team, the Portsmouth Cubs. While in seminary he was ordained a Methodist minister and served rural churches in Chesterfield County, Virginia. Subsequently, he joined the Episcopal Church, was ordained priest, and served congregations in Newport News, Virginia, and Knoxville, Tennessee. He holds an M.Div. from Presbyterian Theological Seminary, in Richmond; an S.T.M. from the School of Theology, University of the South; and a D. Min. from New York Theological Seminary. He did two years of post-graduate studies at the University of St. Andrews in Scotland and at Mansfield College, Oxford University in England. He completed two years of clinical training in residencies at St. Luke's Episcopal Texas Children's Hospital, in Houston, and at Central State Hospital, in Milledgeville, Georgia.

His life's work has been principally in the field of clinical pastoral care and counseling and pastoral psychotherapy. He was certified clinical supervisor by the Association for Clinical Pastoral Education in 1970 and held leadership positions with that organization. In 1988, he began publishing the *ACPE Underground Report*, which later morphed into *Contra Mundum*. In 1990, with colleagues, he founded the College of Pastoral Supervision and Psychotherapy and has served as its General Secretary since. His last position was for 15 years as Director of Pastoral Care, New York Presbyterian Hospital, and Columbia-Presbyterian Medical Center in New York City.

Lawrence has published widely in the fields of social ethics, sexuality, and religion. His articles have appeared in the *Journal of the American Medical Association (JAMA)*, *Annals of Behavioral Medicine*, *Journal of Religion and Health*, *Journal of Pastoral Care and Counseling*, *The Christian Century*, and others. His opinions have appeared in *The New York Times*, *The Washington Post*, *Los Angeles Times*, *The Dallas Morning News* and a number of other newspapers. He is the author of four books: *The Poisoning of Eros: Sexual Values in Conflict; Sexual Liberation: The Scandal of Christendom; Nine Clinical Cases: The Soul of Pastoral Care and Counseling;* and *Recovery of Soul: A History and Memoir of the Clinical Pastoral Movement*. He is an amateur mycologist, founder of the Texas Mycological Society, and a lover of baseball. He may be reached at lawrence@cpsp.org.

www.ingramcontent.com/pod-product-compliance
Lightning Source LLC
Chambersburg PA
CBHW021144160426
43194CB00007B/678